SOCIAL PSYCHIATRY

TAVISTOCK

The International Behavioural and Social Sciences Library

PSYCHIATRY
In 5 Volumes

SOCIAL PSYCHIATRY

A Study of Therapeutic Communities

MAXWELL JONES
AND A BAKER, THOMAS FREEMAN,
JULIUS MERRY, B A POMRYN, JOSEPH
SANDLER AND JOY TUXFORD

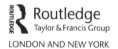

Routledge
Taylor & Francis Group

LONDON AND NEW YORK

First published in 1952 by
Tavistock Publications Limited

Reprinted in 2001 by
Routledge
2 Park Square, Milton Park, Abingdon, Oxon, OX14 4RN

Simultaneously published in the USA and Canada by Routledge
711 Third Avenue, New York, NY 10017

Transferred to Digital Printing 2007

Routledge is an imprint of the Taylor & Francis Group, an informa business

First issued in paperback 2013

The publishers have made every effort to contact authors/copyright holders
of the works reprinted in the *International Behavioural and Social Sciences
Library*. This has not been possible in every case, however, and we would
welcome correspondence from those individuals/companies we have been
unable to trace.

These reprints are taken from original copies of each book. In many cases
the condition of these originals is not perfect. The publisher has gone to
great lengths to ensure the quality of these reprints, but wishes to point
out that certain characteristics of the original copies will, of necessity, be
apparent in reprints thereof.

British Library Cataloguing in Publication Data
A CIP catalogue record for this book
is available from the British Library

Social Psychiatry

ISBN 978-0-415-26476-1 (hbk)
ISBN 978-0-415-86599-9 (pbk)

SOCIAL PSYCHIATRY

A Study of Therapeutic Communities

by

MAXWELL JONES

M.D., M.R.C.P.(EDIN.), D.P.M.

and

A. BAKER, M.B., B.S., D.P.M.

THOMAS FREEMAN, M.D., D.P.M.

JULIUS MERRY, M.B., B.S., D.P.M.

B. A. POMRYN, M.B., B.S., D.P.M.

JOSEPH SANDLER, M.A., Ph.D., A.I.S.

JOY TUXFORD

with a foreword by

PROFESSOR AUBREY LEWIS

TAVISTOCK PUBLICATIONS LIMITED

First published in 1952
by Tavistock Publications Limited
in collaboration with
Routledge
2 Park Square, Milton Park, Abingdon,
Oxon, OX14 4RN

This book is dedicated to
THE NURSING STAFF
*who have formed a framework
around which
our therapeutic communities
have been built*

FOREWORD

THE insistent needs and the aspirations of the last war gave a vigorous impetus to social measures in every sphere. This was true of medicine in all its divisions, and notably so in psychiatry which by its nature is a field of social knowledge and practice. The studies undertaken in war-time and the bold experiments made were for the most part not so much new in theoretical outlook or method as ambitious and flexible, with the wider scope made possible by the circumstances of the time. Many of these psychiatric efforts, like those in other branches of medicine, have taken on a different proportion during the ensuing years, some growing and changing, others dwindling. Among the most lasting is the still developing experiment described in this book by Dr. Maxwell Jones and his associates.

Dr. Maxwell Jones was well equipped by his previous training for the physiological and clinical studies which he pursued during his charge of the Effort Syndrome Unit at Mill Hill. These were objective inquiries, rigorously executed. But for the socially directed work which began during that period and is here set out, he was less well prepared, for he had had no contact with the social investigations of other psychiatrists, and his interests in treatment were mainly concerned with the highly individual approach derived from psychoanalysis. Transfer of training is a debated question in psychology; it will, however, be clear to anyone who reads the book that Dr. Maxwell Jones has carried over much of his earlier scientific training and experience to the conduct of the experiment in which he has put all his energies for the last few years, and to its use for research. Chapters VIII and IX testify to that. But faith and zeal are effective in carrying through a pioneer social venture when habits of objective verification and severe stage-by-stage appraisal would impose delays or be out of keeping with the aims of the project. Dr. Maxwell Jones wanted to take the tide at the flood, in the post-war period when the

Ministry of Labour and public opinion were favourable to the task of 'social engineering' he had set himself. He has demonstrated the effect of such a therapeutic community as he developed at Belmont, upon the mental health and occupational fitness of men whose character and medical history augured badly in these regards. What he has not demonstrated so clearly, though it can be inferred from what he has accomplished and is known to those in touch with his work, is the unremitting energy, sustained purpose and enthusiasm which he has put into this difficult enterprise. To these qualities and his judgment and experience it chiefly owes the success of which this book gives evidence.

AUBREY LEWIS

University of London   *Professor of Psychiatry*

ACKNOWLEDGEMENTS

THE authors wish to acknowledge the collaboration of Miss Elizabeth Cann, Miss Molly Chennell, Mr. M. Desai, M.A., B.Com., Ll.B., Ph.D., and Mr. W. B. Shaw.

We wish to thank Dr. Louis Minski, Physician Superintendent of Belmont Hospital for his friendly and helpful attitude towards this experiment.

We also wish to thank various members of the Ministry of Labour who have collaborated with us. They have shown a remarkable appreciation of the needs of the disabled person and have never failed to meet our requests for help in a most competent manner.

Numerous doctors have been on our staff during the period of our experiment and have all contributed to the work; they include Drs. E. D. Barlow, D. H. Bennett, M. Wilks, J. L. Rowley, B. Shorvon, J. Styrt and A. S. Thorley.

Sister Maureen Chivers participated in all three therapeutic communities and made a unique contribution.

Finally, we would like to thank the local communities of Dartford (Kent) and Sutton (Surrey) for their pioneer spirit in trying to help to rehabilitate hospital patients.

CONTENTS

INTRODUCTION

THIS book is a report on the work of a unit which was organized to study and develop community methods of treatment. Many different factors led to its inception. The inquiry really started ten years ago when a trend towards group treatment and studies of the patient community appeared in British psychiatry; these trends were developed by Army psychiatrists and psychologists and by the Emergency Medical Service of the Ministry of Health; the experiments at Mill Hill and Dartford (both Ministry of Health hospitals) which are briefly described in this book, were forerunners of the present Industrial Neurosis Unit at Belmont Hospital which was started in April 1947.

The development of community methods of treatment implies the wider application of the social sciences, mainly sociology and anthropology, to existing psychiatric practice. War-time needs with the huge volume of psychiatric cases and relative shortage of psychiatrists gave a tremendous stimulus to social methods of treatment in psychiatry; but probably more important is the changing cultural pattern in Britain. It appears to us that, in this country at least, the community is to-day assuming social responsibilities which would not have been contemplated a generation ago. This growth of a social conscience goes much deeper than the political changes which have occurred during recent years, although these are themselves a manifestation of social change. A good illustration of this change in the climate of opinion is the Disabled Persons (Employment) Act of 1944. This Act was designed to protect the interests of the disabled person in the employment field. In this Act the expression 'disabled person' means a person who, on account of injury, disease (physically or psychologically determined), or congenital deformity, is substantially handicapped in obtaining or keeping employment, or in undertaking work on his own account of a kind which, apart from his disability, would be suited to his age, experience, and qualifications. To implement the Act a considerable social machinery has been established under the Ministry of Labour which aims at obtaining the optimum conditions of work in open or sheltered employment for every disabled person capable of some form of employment. This means a substantial expenditure of time and money by the Government. The fact that at present Britain is a country with full employment does of course aid such legislation, and the climate of opinion might well change with the development of unemployment. My point is that, given certain social conditions, a nation has demonstrated its willingness to assume responsibility and strive to obtain optimal working conditions for its less functionally useful members.

I think that this same development of a social consciousness has resulted in the establishment of neurosis centres in this country; a generation ago our patients would have been assailed with much good advice by their friends, or ordered to 'pull themselves together', or have drifted into a work-house. Nowadays these patients are regarded as psychological casualties in the struggles of everyday life, who may need a special hospital environment in order to have their problems investigated and, if possible, dealt with. The Industrial Neurosis Unit at Belmont Hospital is a further extension of this trend; not only is psychiatric treatment attempted but a serious attempt at resettlement is made. We admit from all parts of the country patients who have long-standing neuroses and character disorders, and have also employment difficulties. Officially the Unit has the backing of three Government Ministries—those of Health, Labour, and Pensions. Thus we have a strong positive sanction from above; without this sanction a unit such as the one at Belmont could hardly survive. It is filled with patients who include some of the most anti-social elements in society—people who have served prison sentences, drug addicts, prostitutes, and so on; the fact that they are the symptoms of a sick society may arouse fear and anger in the larger community, as well as the social consciousness which I have been discussing. Clearly we have forced on us a tremendous responsibility not only in regard to treatment in the usual psychiatric sense, but also from the sociological point of view. These patients frequently exert a strong negative influence on the environment from which they come, and if treatment in hospital is relatively unsuccessful, as is all too frequently the case, then disposal presents great difficulties. For instance, is it wise to place some man with a severe character disorder in a job where he may disrupt the existing community? Considerations like this, plus the unsuitability of this type of chronic neurotic and character disorder for short-term methods of psychiatric treatment, have underlined the necessity for experimentation with community methods of treatment. Our patients represent the 'failures' in society; they come largely from broken homes and are unemployed; inevitably they have developed anti-social attitudes in an attempt to defend themselves from what appears to them as a hostile environment; as often as not their marriages are in ruins and there is little or no attempt to keep up any of the more usual standards of behaviour in their home life. They are out of work and this absence of a work role leads almost inevitably to a disruption of the man's social relationships. To bring cases of this 'hopeless' kind together into one hospital must lead to chaos or worse unless there is a well-defined social structure and a well-trained staff to maintain this structure. How this is attempted is described in the following chapters. Briefly we attempt to absorb the patient into the Unit community, which has developed a definite culture of its own. This culture is a fairly sophisticated one and is maintained and perpetuated through the staff rather than through the patients, although in practice it is difficult to separate these two groups in the Unit community. Educational techniques, mainly in the form of discussion groups, seem to aid any change in social attitudes in the desocialized patient. As far as possible social and vocational roles are provided for him while still in hospital, and employment in the outside community is sometimes preferable to the more restricted hospital workshops. These roles approximate as far as possible to what is found in the relatively healthy outside community; thus the workshops attempt to simulate ordinary factory conditions and there is none of the individual diversionary aim commonly associated with occupational therapy in hospital. That social attitudes can be made to change by means of such community techniques has been shown by the 'follow-up study'.

Rehabilitation and resettlement work is carried out in this country mainly by the Ministries of Health and Labour; to a smaller extent it is done by the Ministry of Pensions, and various charitable organizations. The biggest organization at the present time is that which has developed under the Ministry of Labour who have been in this field since 1941; at that time the shortage of manpower for the Armed Forces and for industry led to greater attempts to use the disabled population as a source of further manpower. It soon became clear that the disabled man could be absorbed in industry with advantage to both in most cases. This led up to the passing of the Disabled Persons (Employment) Act in 1944. This Act was designed to protect the interests of the disabled person in the employment field, and where necessary or practicable to set up sheltered conditions of employment; it also made provision for various forms of training. All employers in this country with more than twenty employees are required to employ 3 per cent of disabled persons.

The Ministry of Labour keeps a register of disabled persons; the applicant must satisfy the Ministry that he is in fact disabled, and that his disablement is likely to continue for six months or more. The total number of registered disabled persons in Britain at the beginning of 1950 was just under one million (936,196). Of these 40.7 per cent were classed as surgical; 37.5 per cent as medical; 5.2 per cent as psychiatric; and miscellaneous 16.6 per cent. There is little doubt that with more careful scrutiny the psychiatric group would be greatly increased. Of the registered disabled persons 65,128 were unemployed in April 1950, and of these approximately 8 per cent were classified as 'psychiatric'. Of the 65,128 unemployed disabled persons, 9,623 were classified as unlikely to obtain employment except under sheltered conditions.

The disabled person is interviewed in private at the Ministry of Labour Employment Exchanges by Disablement Resettlement Officers (D.R.O.s). In January 1950 there were 366 full-time and 1,450 part-time D.R.O.s in the United Kingdom. For the year ended 31st January 1950, the total placings in Britain of unemployed registered disabled persons by the D.R.O.s was 214,586 persons—a monthly average of 17,883.

In order to assist the Ministry of Labour in the resettlement of cases presenting special problems, twelve Industrial Rehabilitation Units (I.R.U.s) have been set up in the big cities in Britain. These units are attached to existing Government training centres, and have factory-like conditions in the workshops. They take approximately one hundred men at a time for periods of six to eight weeks. The units are non-residential and an adult man is paid a maintenance allowance of seventy shillings a week if single, and eighty shillings a week if married. The intake is drawn mainly from general hospitals and Health Service doctors who send patients no longer needing active medical treatment, but who are not yet ready for full employment. The other main source of intake is from the unemployed disabled persons and these are referred by the D.R.O.s. At the centre the disabled man is frequently employed on actual production work, each I.R.U. being left free to develop its own contacts with local industry in the form of sub-contracts and so on. The staff of the I.R.U. includes a rehabilitation officer selected for his industrial experience and administrative ability; other members of the team are a vocational guidance officer, a social worker, a D.R.O., a chief occupational supervisor and a doctor. The latter is chosen for his interest in resettlement work and preferably has some previous experience of industrial work or social medicine. Since the opening of the centres in 1948, 8,607 people had been admitted up to May 1950. So far over 80 per cent of persons have been found employment or been placed in training. In addition to the I.R.U.s the Government has established over eighty factories called Remploy factories for sheltered employment. These are administered by a special corporation and take an average of one hundred disabled persons each. These people would be quite unable to maintain employment under normal working conditions—e.g. they include severe orthopaedic deformities, advanced cases of disseminated sclerosis, cardiac disease, severe epileptics and so on. In the main they are working on Government contracts and so far no trouble has arisen over competition with private enterprise. They make such things as furniture and violins for the Ministry of Education, surgical boots for the Ministry of Health, and miners' gloves for the National Coal Board. Pay is, by agreements with the unions, slightly less than the standard trade-union rate.

To aid the Ministry of Labour in carrying out their function in the disablement field, a National Advisory Council on the Employment of the Disabled has been formed. It includes representatives from employers' organizations, trade unions, representatives from the various benevolent societies, Government officials, and four doctors. As a member of this Council I have been particularly interested in the vast sociological implications of the Disabled Persons (Employment) Act. The most troublesome aspect of the problem, from the point of view of the Council, probably centres around the 'hard core' of chronic unemployed persons. They take up a large part of the D.R.O.s' time at the employment exchanges, and, although a relatively small group, are enormously important sociologically. Whatever the diagnostic label attached to these people may be, their unemployment and failure to compensate for their disability leads to various anti-social attitudes, and in this sense they become psychiatric problems. The Industrial Neurosis Unit at Belmont is an attempt to examine a sample of this population and investigate various methods of treatment and resettlement. Our experience has been useful in planning the development of the Ministry of Labour Industrial Rehabilitation Units already referred to. In the 'Second Report of the Standing Committee on the Rehabilitation and Resettlement of Disabled Persons' (London, H.M. Stationery Office, 1949), this is alluded to in paragraph 21 as follows:

'The work of this Unit (Belmont) is regarded as a social experiment and is closely related to the whole problem of unemployment among disabled persons. The experience gained is being used in planning non-residential centres (Industrial Resettlement Units) . . . which are being established in various industrial areas.'

The close contact with the national problem of resettlement of disabled persons through the Ministry of Labour and the National Advisory Council on the Employment of the Disabled, has given a vital stimulus to the work at Belmont. Dealing with this type of chronic neurotic unemployed individual can be both depressing and disheartening. The knowledge that information in this field was badly needed for the satisfactory implementation of the Disabled Persons (Employment) Act, however, offset discouragement which might otherwise have crept in. Along with this has been the growing conviction amongst the staff community that much could be done to improve the lot of the chronic neurotic by social methods of treatment. We have gained enormously by our own social structure which has afforded opportunity for discussion of our emotional problems and group tensions. The staff, and to some extent the patients, have felt that they have participated in a creative experiment and this has been helped by frequent contact with visitors from the social science field. Visitors are welcomed every Friday morning from 9 a.m. to 12 noon during which time they see a psychodrama, visit the workshops, and sit in at a placement conference. We have had approximately 400 visitors in the last year, and wherever possible the entire Unit staff has been present. In this way visitors, far from being an inconvenience, have helped us greatly and kept us in contact with outside world opinion in the rehabilitation sphere.

I have been fortunate in having the opportunity to study rehabilitation procedures in many countries while working as a consultant in mental health to the World Health Organization. A report, 'Rehabilitation in Psychiatry', is in progress.

In conclusion I would like to say that this work would have been quite impossible but for the unusually stable and loyal staff on the Unit. Work in this sphere seems to bring out the best in people and in preparing this book I am very conscious of the fact that I am no more than an articulate member of a highly integrated group.

CHAPTER I

TWO EARLY EXPERIMENTAL COMMUNITIES

I. THE EFFORT SYNDROME UNIT AT MILL HILL EMERGENCY HOSPITAL

D URING the war years Mill Hill Public School was used as a
psychiatric centre run by the Ministry of Health. The staff was
drawn from the Maudsley Hospital which had been closed at
the outbreak of war. The hospital was situated in beautiful grounds on
the northern outskirts of London. A second team from the Maudsley
Hospital was set up at Sutton on the southern fringe of London.
These two neurosis centres, although springing from the same parent
body, developed along very different lines. Sutton Emergency Hospital came to be associated with short-term methods of treatment
which proved particularly effective with the more acute forms of
war neuroses, and such techniques as modified insulin, ether abreaction, continuous narcosis, and narcoanalysis were employed on a
large scale there. The work at Mill Hill followed very different lines.
There the emphasis lay in the application of sociological and psychological concepts to treatment.

An effort syndrome unit of 100 beds was set up at Mill Hill under
the joint directorship of a cardiologist (Paul Wood) and a psychiatrist
(M.J.); the former remained on the staff for eighteen months and his
highly informative study of the problem of effort syndrome (neurocirculatory asthenia) was published in his Goulstonion Lectures.[1] For
the remaining three and a half years of the war I was entirely responsible for the running of the Effort Syndrome Unit and was given almost unlimited freedom by the Medical Superintendent, Dr. The
Hon. W. S. Maclay. To start with, the wards were indistinguishable
from those of a general hospital ward, with a large ambulant population. The nurse's role was not clearly defined but her traditions were
largely those of the general hospital nurse. The Sister's (charge

[1] Paul Wood, *Brit. med. J.*, 1, 767, 805, 845 (1941).

nurse's) word was law and very little free communication existed between nurse and doctor, and nurse and patient. At this time we were getting an excellent type of girl to do temporary war-time nursing. These were often educated mature women from the professions who chose to do nursing as their war work. (In Britain conscription was compulsory for women to almost the extent that applied in the case of men.) Clearly such people expected and deserved an active role in the treatment programme. At the same time, the temporary war-time nature of the nursing staff, and indeed of the hospital, afforded the opportunity to develop a type of nursing training appropriate to a neurosis hospital alongside the formal training essential to those of our nurses who wished to achieve official status through the only State examination available to them. In other words every use was made of the opportunity to train nurses for the work of the hospital rather than for the role of the mental nurse which had little bearing on our own particular needs but which gave them status, better pay and security. The trend was more and more towards the tutorial system and integration of the work of the doctors and nurses. Inevitably a change occurred in the social structure of the ward. The Sister ceased to be a liaison between the other nurses and the doctor and free direct communication between those two groups was encouraged; in the same way the nurse was expected to communicate freely with the patient and came to play a leader role, e.g. she frequently kept a ward log book where the fourteen patients in her ward recorded some of the problems affecting the group, and described how these problems were met through discussion. These early changes in the community structure threw a considerable strain on the Ward Sister who felt that her authority was being undermined; in fact the whole development almost broke down as a result of the anxiety aroused in the senior nursing group. Luckily the Medical Superintendent and Matron supported the reform and without this sanction the development would have had to be postponed.

Along with the foregoing changes in the staff community there were important changes occurring in the patient group. The patients were made up entirely of Service personnel suffering from effort syndrome; this meant that their symptomatology was almost identical. They complained of breathlessness, palpitations, left chest pain, postural giddiness, occasional fainting attacks and fatigue; their symptoms were in the main related to exercise. To begin with the problem was considered to be one calling for careful inquiry into each individual case and a full physical (cardiological) and psychiatric examination. In addition extensive physiological researches were carried out in continuation of the work done in this field by Sir Thomas Lewis and his collaborators in the First World War.[1, 2, 3] As a result of these inquiries much factual data were accumulated, e.g. we found that prolonged tension in certain muscles (apparently a peripheral manifestation of anxiety) accounted for some of the symptoms found in effort syndrome. The diaphragmatic movement was measured on the x-ray screen and found to be restricted towards the inspiratory end of respiration; this resulted in the rapid shallow breathing so characteristic of patients with effort syndrome. Those patients complaining of left chest pain showed on screening the greatest degree of restriction of diaphragmatic movement; the left chest pain was apparently due to an associated tension and fatigue in the diaphragmatic and intercostal muscles which were frequently tender to the touch; this pain could be abolished by an injection of novacain into the affected muscles or by a root block (Paul Wood). We demonstrated that these patients used up more oxygen in doing a known amount of work than did normal controls; also that when worked to exhaustion on a bicycle ergometer they had a significantly lower blood lacate than normal controls, i.e. they appeared to give up at a 'non-physiological' end point, presumably due to fear of the harmful effects of exercise on their supposedly weak hearts. As the understanding of individual symptoms developed it became clear that effort syndrome was a psychosomatic complaint and whatever might be the individual psychological contributory factors, the peripheral mechanisms were much the same in each case. This being so it seemed reasonable to explain to the patients the physiological mechanisms involved in the production of symptoms. To do this to each of the 100 patients in the ward individually would have taken many hundreds of hours and been monotonously repetitive. A start was made in discussing at a mechanistic level the meaning of symptoms with the whole group of 100 patients. The 'lecture' approach was soon abandoned and a discussion procedure adopted.

It was found necessary to give the patients a certain amount of instruction in elementary physiology and anatomy in order that they

[1] Lewis, T., *The Soldier's Heart and the Effort Syndrome*. London. Shaw.
[2] Paul Wood, *Brit. Med. J.*, 1, 767, 805, 845 (1941).
[3] Jones, M., *Jour. Ment. Sc.*, 94, 392, Apr. 1948.

should understand the nature of their symptoms. We decided eventually that at least twelve hours of discussion and instruction were needed for our purpose. Meetings were held three times a week for a month and the course then repeated. The average length of a patient's stay in hospital was six to eight weeks so that there were always men in the ward who had had a complete course. In time it became possible to conduct the discussion group in such a way that the information required was obtained almost entirely from the audience. This had particular value in war-time when soldiers in general, and neurotic soldiers in particular, were always on guard against being 'got at' by those in authority. It was enough to set the group a problem, e.g. the mechanisms involved in breathlessness and left chest pain, and merely to direct the discussion which then followed. In this way the patients were kept interested and readily accepted the information offered by their more informed fellow-patients. It must be remembered that we were dealing with a young adult male population who were in the main mechanistically inclined; they were helped considerably by life-size diagrams of the nervous system, etc., painted by one of the nurses, and by a model brain. A patient who was a journalist kindly took down a verbatim account of a complete series of these twelve talks. Two meetings are reported here and these have not been in any way altered for publication.

Meeting 6. Wed. December 15th, 1943.
Last week we talked about fear. What did we decide about it?
A PATIENT: It is a useful spur.
What else?
A PATIENT: A stimulant.
Yes.
A PATIENT: A protection.
Yes. We decided that it was a normal and useful thing at times but that at other times it was useless. Give me an illustration of when it is not useful.
A PATIENT: In times of personal disaster.
Yes. So far we have considered the voluntary nervous system, the thinking part of the brain which receives the messages from the outside world and controls movements and behaviour. Then we considered the control room, the headquarters of the involuntary nervous system, and the involuntary nervous system itself which does what?

A PATIENT: Regulates the functions of the body.

Yes. It regulates the working of the organs, of the blood supply, digesting food and so on. They are all regulated for you. If you had to regulate them yourselves you would make a hash of it. We have considered these in normal health and now we are beginning to consider the other side. Fear is the introduction to the next phase which is the nervous system when it is upset and it is necessary for us to consider what we mean by calling anyone nervous. What do we mean?

A PATIENT: He has lost his equilibrium.

A PATIENT: Circumstances make one rather different from what one normally is, when one is excited.

I don't quite know what you mean by that. What do you mean by excited?

A PATIENT: In an hysterical condition as shown by your reaction to various circumstances.

A PATIENT: Not in harmony with the circumstances.

Yes. Do you mean internal or external harmony?

A PATIENT: The spark between the voluntary and involuntary nervous systems is missing.

Just picture a nervous man—someone obviously suffering from a nervous condition. What makes you think he is nervous?

A PATIENT: By his actions and the way he speaks—his reaction to circumstances—lack of control.

When he loses control what else do you note?

A PATIENT: His body shakes.

What else?

A PATIENT: He loses his interest in life.

Yes. People who are interested in life notice all sorts of things. It is a question of using your eyes and seeing things.

A PATIENT: Well, he goes white. He is shy. His muscles are tense. His eyes have a sheepish look about them or a look of fear. The pupils of the eyes would dilate.

What about the size of the eyes?

A PATIENT: I don't think you would notice anything about the eyes.

I can't agree with that. Stand opposite someone and make a loud noise and you will see a dilation of the eyes. What does Eddie Cantor look like? Startled. Doesn't that suggest fear? Surprise has an element of fear in it. These are some of the things that make you think a person is nervous. Cold and clammy hands, too, are a definite indication of nervousness. They show that there is a poor circulation which usually goes with nervousness. All these things have something in common. What is it?

A PATIENT: The involuntary nervous system is wrong.

In what way?

A PATIENT: Due to lack of co-ordination.

Yes. The individual has some disturbance which interferes with the normal functioning of the involuntary nervous system. This is a complicated and interesting phenomenon and if a 'superior' person, in the lay sense, when he talks of 'nervousness', really knew he was describing a very complex psychological happening, he would not feel so 'superior'. Let us give an explanation of what causes nervousness. We are interested in harmony from the point of view of our own lives and also as a study of the involuntary nervous system. Can you widen the description?

A PATIENT: Physical and mental reaction to the outside.

A PATIENT: Disharmony of the nervous system caused by a disturbance of the mental state by some disturbance of the brain.

What part of the brain?

A PATIENT: A conflict in the conscious brain affecting the involuntary nerves. External disharmony mirrored by internal disharmony.

Give an illustration of how it works.

A PATIENT: Well, you get it in a person's dislike for crowds.

Yes, take something simpler.

A PATIENT: If we hear a loud bang the sound is carried through our ears and we receive an impression through our voluntary nervous system and if we cannot do anything about it our involuntary nervous system will get us ready to run or something like that.

Yes. A loud explosion would have a response which would put everything in readiness for action. The explosion has disturbed the external harmony. Suppose you are walking down the street and a car back-fires or a child is run over—you get disharmony, a state of mental conflict which upsets you, makes you turn pale and so on. Changes occur in the involuntary nervous system which make you nervous and you may remain in that state for the rest of the day. You are jumpy. You lose your appetite. The impression of the accident lingers and you have a state of nervousness.

A PATIENT: How can you counteract that?

You can't. It is perfectly natural. We are working through from the normal to the abnormal. Our definition of nervousness is now what?

A PATIENT: Disturbances set up in the voluntary and involuntary nervous systems.

Yes. You could be a bit more informative, couldn't you?

A PATIENT: The two systems are not working in harmony.

Yes. Nervousness is a condition actuated by fear which produces a disharmony in the two systems—from the voluntary nervous system to the involuntary nervous system. An accident, or something of that kind causes a disturbance in the voluntary part of the brain. This is reflected in a disturbance in the normal smooth working of the involuntary part of the nervous system which controls the organs of the body and leads to disharmony. When you talk of someone being nervous, you mean something quite elaborate. The disturbances of the involuntary nervous system can be understood in a more detailed or mechanical way. Here is a chart showing the double nerve supply to each organ. Why is there a double supply?

A PATIENT: One speeds up the impulses, and the other retards them.

Yes. One is the accelerator and the other the brake. When a nerve is stimulated what happens? Some of you can think in terms of electrical frequencies which can be measured. If you were studying what is happening from a more detailed point of view, how would you measure it?

A PATIENT: You would need some sort of a meter.

What sort of a meter? You could put a fine platinum wire into part of the nerve and another into another part, and fix a galvonometer in the circuit. You could put a galvonometer in the nerve itself, or into a muscle—it would not really matter which because the current is going to cause contraction of the muscle in any case. As the muscle contracts, the vibration is increased, and when it relaxes it slows down so that you can measure the degree of nervousness in a person. I want you to realize quite pictorially that nervousness can be measured.

What do you mean when you say a person is tense?

A PATIENT: His muscles are tense.

Yes.

A PATIENT: Because he is excited.

What do you mean by excited?

A PATIENT: His nerves are stimulated.

Yes, they are more reactive or responsive. This is not a vague conception but a very accurate one, and it can be measured. So when you talk about a person being nervous you mean that his muscles are tense. You can narrow down your description of nervousness to one of muscle tenseness. Which muscles?

A PATIENT: The face muscles, legs, hands, and arms. (Yes, people frequently clasp their hands when they are nervous.) The diaphragm.

Yes, what does it do?

A PATIENT: It contracts.

Yes, how?

A PATIENT: Upwards.

No, it would go down when it contracted. What other muscles?

A PATIENT: The bladder. The stomach.

Yes, your stomach stops working and 'turns over' if you hear a bomb drop. It contracts.

A PATIENT: The neck muscles also contract.

Yes, every muscle you can think of contracts when you are tense. Are there any muscles we have left out?

A PATIENT: The heart.

Yes. What do you notice about the skin or the hair?

A PATIENT: The hair stands upright.

Why?

A PATIENT: Contraction of the muscles of the scalp.

That is what you mean by nervousness or muscle-tension. Nervousness is perfectly easily understood, and it can be worked out as a state of disturbance of the involuntary nervous system.

Meeting 8. Monday December 20th, 1943.

What did we cover last time?

A PATIENT: Relaxation.

Yes. Any particular aspect of it?

A PATIENT: How to overcome tenseness?

Yes. Why did we choose tenseness?

A PATIENT: Because it is the state into which the muscles get when we are actuated by fear.

Yes. We defined what we meant by nervousness, and we decided that nervous tension and muscle tension were much the same thing. We decided there were two ways of coping with nervousness. What were they?

A PATIENT: Relaxation was one way, and the brain was the other.

Yes. You can tackle the trouble at its source or at the symptoms. Where do we tackle the problem?

A PATIENT: If your muscles are tense and you are worried, try to think of something else, and that will give you relaxation.

No. That would be side-stepping it. When we talk about relaxation we mean the muscles. By an effort of will you can try to bring about relaxation by concentrating on the muscles that are tense. If you are tense you should try to get comfortable and relax. I saw a very intelligent man a few days ago who has a very bad stammer, and he had worked it out for himself. He was very anxious to get treatment. He was prepared to pay for treatment which is a very good thing; you appreciate treatment if you pay for it, and this is one reason why doctors like to have fees—so that the patient will think it is important. This fellow had studied his stammer, and he was conscious of the fact that when he began to speak he got a feeling of tenseness in the region of the diaphragm. He discovered that if at these times he sat in a certain position, his stammer was better. He made a point of getting really comfortable and loosening up, and his stammer was really much better. This is an application of the principle of muscle tension and muscle relaxation. This morning our goal is an understanding of two things—breathlessness and left chest pain. What is the explanation of breathlessness? Are you people more breathless than the soldiers from the local barracks?

A PATIENT: Yes.

Let's work it out in a logical way. What is the first important thing that contributes to your breathlessness?

A PATIENT: You are not physically fit.

In what sense?

A PATIENT: The muscles are tense.

Yes. Why do you get more breathless? Work it out. The diaphragm is shaped something like a bell-tent, and is fixed at the bottom. It is moving. It is like a muscular dome and the dome moves upwards. When it contracts it flattens out, and as it relaxes it comes up again. What does your diaphragm do when you take a deep breath?

A PATIENT: It flattens.

Is there more space or less?

A PATIENT: More space, I suppose.

So what happens? When you take a breath there is less space below. Everything is squeezed up. How does it make more room?

A PATIENT: Your stomach expands.

Yes. It bulges. The abdominal contents are forced down, and they tend to bulge. At the same time your chest wall goes up. The movement of the ribs and contraction of the diaphragm make more room, and the air is sucked in. That is normal health. Why are you people more breathless than the average person?

A PATIENT: I suppose the nervous system accounts for it. The muscles don't do their job properly, and as a result you can't breathe properly.

What is the exact mechanism of your breathlessness?

A PATIENT: The muscles of the diaphragm contract, and instead of a regular up and down motion, they vibrate.

No. Not altogether. That is a bit of drama of your own. You are quite right, but don't bring in vibration. If your diaphragm is taut instead of having a free movement, what is the effect on your breathing? Your breathing is not as deep as it should be. You get shallower and more rapid breathing, and the tautness of the muscles of the chest wall will have the same effect. You tend to breathe with your diaphragm down. You are breathing with just a small movement of the diaphragm and your chest muscles are taut, and your chest is inclined to be up. The diaphragm tends to contract. If you are nervous the movement is considerably cut down.

If you heard a bomb coming down, what would happen?

A PATIENT: The diaphragm would contract.

Yes. The diaphragm would just stop working, and go into a spasm. The same thing would happen if you jumped into a swimming pool. The diaphragm would contract down, and your chest would go up.

A PATIENT: The tendency is always to take a deep breath on the spur of the moment.

Would you expect your breathing to be more rapid than that of other people?

A PATIENT: It depends on the individual.

Even when asleep you people breathe more rapidly than others. The muscle tension is still there. Patients in this hospital breathe at twice the rate of the ordinary population. What about the depth of your breathing?

A PATIENT: It is shallower.

Yes. To what extent?

A PATIENT: Half.

Yes. You really get as much oxygen as anyone else, but you make more fuss and bother about it. You are doing more work to get the same amount of oxygen. Now what about this left chest pain? What causes this pain in the chest?

A PATIENT: Over-exertion.

How does over-exertion cause it?

A PATIENT: You might have a weak heart.

You ought to be 'scalped'. It is a crime to talk about a weak heart here. What causes the pain?

A PATIENT: I should think it is in the left chest because it might have something to do with the arteries leading to the heart.

What causes the pain?

A PATIENT: The muscles. They are not contracting to the full extent.

The muscles begin to ache because they are working overtime. Is that reasonable? Could you cause the same pain in some other muscle?

A PATIENT: Yes. In your arm.

Yes. If you are reading and hold a book for a long time, your arm begins to ache. What sort of pain do most of you get?

A PATIENT: A dull ache, or a sharp stab.

Is the dull ache any different from the ache you would get in your arm?

A PATIENT: No.

That is right. It is the same sort of pain. Have any of you had lumbago? Is the short stabbing pain of lumbago the same as the pain you get in your chest?

A PATIENT: Yes.

How can we prove that this pain is a muscle pain?

A PATIENT: By an injection into the muscle—something to make the muscles relax.

Well that it reasonable, but the trouble is that you have to keep on breathing. You don't want to stop for a day or two. What exactly would you do with the muscles? Inject them with what?

A PATIENT: Some sort of anaesthetic to kill the pain. If the pain is coming from the muscles, it should then stop.

Would you accept this as absolute proof?

A PATIENT: Yes.

That is what we used to do here. It is deep down, about two inches or so. If you inject deep into these muscles you put away the pain. We have done it. Of course the pain comes back after the anaesthetic has worn off. There is no possible doubt that the pain is muscle pain, and that it comes from overworking these muscles. Why the left side, and not the right side as a rule?

A PATIENT: Because the heart is the main muscle.

But the pain isn't coming from the heart? Which side do you like to sleep on?

A PATIENT: The right side.

Why do you lie on the right side?

A PATIENT: To relieve some sort of pressure from the heart.

By lying on the left side you bring the heart up against the ribs. When I examine you I get you to lie on your left side so that the heart is brought up against the ribs, and I can hear it pumping better. The dull ache is fatigue from overworking the muscles, and the short stabbing pain is a further stage when the nerve ends are sensitive. Breathlessness and left chest pain have much in common, and frequently go together. That is why you people have breathlessness and left chest pain, and it is frequently mistaken for heart disease, although it has nothing at all to do with the heart. When you have heart disease you don't get pain in that position. It is an entirely different type of pain.

The important lesson that emerged from this stage of our work was that by an educational technique a group of 100 patients with similar symptomatology could alter their attitudes towards their symptoms. In the majority of patients the symptoms did not disappear but a fundamental change was effected in the patient's attitude towards his symptoms. On admission most patients considered their symptoms to be due to some form of heart disease usually related to the unusual physical stresses to which their Army training had subjected them. They ignored in the main the emotional implications of their war-time vocation and were generally convinced that they had heart disease. The symptoms quite understandably led them to this conclusion; indeed it is difficult to see how any lay person, suffering from pain in the region of the heart, shortness of breath on even mild exertion, palpitation, giddiness, and fainting attacks could fail to come to the conclusion that his heart was in some way affected. No amount of reassurance by even the most eminent cardiologist could be expected to alter this attitude; this experience had been the lot of most of our patients and such reassurance was usually misunderstood. To the patient, reassurance that his heart was sound was meaningless while his symptoms still persisted. He merely felt hurt and misunderstood while it seemed to him that he was being accused of 'imagining' his complaint. Clearly what he needed was a full explanation of the meaning of the symptoms; such an explanation was never attempted and indeed would have been quite impossible in an ordinary consultation, since our experience led us to believe that twelve hours of instruction and discussion were needed to meet the need of the average patient. Through this discussion technique we were able to change the attitude of the majority of patients towards their symptoms; they achieved a degree of objectivity which they had not previously possessed. They began to think of 'a heart' and they were able to conceptualize somatic disfunction. Previously their symptoms had been interpreted as being a result of heart disease, which to the lay person conjures up an image of some relative or friend in a hospital bed in an advanced stage of cardiac decompensation; in this respect the technique aimed at being directly educational.

It soon became evident, however, that the discussion group was more than an educational meeting; it was affecting the whole social structure of the ward. Patients began to use the opportunity afforded by the discussion group to raise problems bearing on the ward life. The group atmosphere was felt to change from day to day sometimes apparently in response to known external stresses, while at other times mysterious unknown forces seemed to be at work. My interest began to widen and question the meaning of the sociological phenomena which occurred within the discussion group. The nurses who attended these meetings began to recognize characteristic patterns of behaviour in their own patients, and became interested in such problems as ward morale. We began to experiment with techniques having a more sociological implication. Social problems were raised for discussion and for a long time the nurses acted out scenes from the lives of a fictitious family comprising the parents (the 'normal' father and hysterical mother) and three daughters whose personalities tended to be schizoid, psychopathic and hysterical respectively. This dramatic approach proved to be tremendously interesting to the patients and provoked a high degree of participation in the subsequent discussion. From here it was only a short step to the patients themselves participating in acting. At first social problems were used and a short play was written on some such theme as alcoholism or illegitimacy. Inevitably the patients writing these short plays projected their own problems into the theme, and it was not long until the appearance of frankly personal presentations occurred in which a patient played his own title role. The use of drama as a technique of social therapy began in January 1944, rapidly became a weekly occurrence and has persisted up to the present time. To begin with we were quite unaware of the work of J. L. Moreno, although latterly we have borrowed freely from his works.

During the war years the social structure of the Effort Syndrome Unit was developing along the lines already indicated. These developments might be summarized under three headings.

1. An attempt was being made to think of treatment as a continuous process operating throughout the entire waking life of the patient while in hospital. The therapeutic interview with the doctor did not alone constitute treatment, while the organization of the rest of the day was being left largely to chance. The patient was reacting to the hospital community in much the same way that he reacted to communities outside. We began to think that a study of these real life situations might be expected to give more information about the nature of the patient's problems, than personal history recounted under the highly artificial conditions of an office interview.

2. In order to make such observation possible, a reorganization of the hospital society was needed with a greater degree of social penetration between the three main sub-groups, patients, nurses and doctors. Thus the original hospital hierarchy was broken down and free communication between doctors, nurses and patients established. The daily discussion between the entire patient population, nurses and doctors and the continuous growth of meetings between various sub-groups, e.g. nurses' tutorials, all aided this process. It is doubtful if the rapid metamorphosis which we witnessed, could have occurred in peacetime; hospital traditions are strong. However, we were helped by the temporary nature of the hospital and of the nurses who were drawn from other professions, together with the general tendency to change which was apparent in many spheres during war-time.

3. Along with the growing awareness of the importance of the communal roles of the doctors and nurses, in addition to their more specific therapeutic functions, the patients' role in the hospital society was being scrutinized. From the early part of the war Dr. Aubrey Lewis had stressed the importance of vocational selection in patients returning to Army duties. The introduction of Army personnel

officers by the Army authorities soon met this need. Considerably less than half of the patients from the Effort Syndrome Unit were discharged from the Army direct from hospital, and despite the favourable labour market which existed during the war, vocational guidance was of great importance with this group if unnecessary stresses in civilian life were to be avoided. To aid the transition from Army to civilian life we began to explore the possibilities of infiltration into the local community, and an arrangement was made with the local technical college to teach type-writing, engineering, etc., to selected groups of patients from Mill Hill Emergency Hospital.

At this stage in our social psychiatric development an exceptional opportunity presented itself for the development of our ideas on community therapeutic techniques. At the beginning of 1945 it was made known to us that the hospital treatment of the most neurotic patients returning from the prisoner-of-war camps in Europe was to be undertaken by a group from Mill Hill Emergency Hospital. Dr. A. B. Stokes who was then Medical Superintendent of the hospital, gave me complete freedom to organize this unit as I thought fit. He himself had a deep interest in social psychiatry and was a member of the National Advisory Council on the Employment of the Disabled which guides the Ministry of Labour in all matters pertaining to the Disabled Persons Act of 1944. During the planning stage Dr. Stokes gave us much invaluable help and many of the ideas put into practice were his. During this planning period, we had an opportunity of studying about twenty ex-prisoners-of-war who had been sent home for medical reasons in accordance with the provisions of the International Red Cross, before the general repatriation began. We made the best possible use of this preliminary experience to plan our hospital organization at the Ex-Prisoner-of-War Unit which was set up at the Southern Hospital, Dartford, Kent, in May 1945.

II. THE EX-PRISONER-OF-WAR UNIT AT THE SOUTHERN HOSPITAL, DARTFORD

This three-hundred bed unit was part of a large general hospital situated in the country near Dartford, a town of thirty-five thousand inhabitants, twenty miles from London. A team of six psychiatrists, fifty nurses, one psychiatric social worker, one occupational instruct-tor and one psychologist, went direct from Mill Hill Emergency Hospital. The Unit was made up of six self-contained blocks each containing fifty beds; most of the cases were referred to us by the Army psychiatrists of the 45th Division who handled the psychiatric problems of the hundred thousand British repatriates from the European theatre.

During the eleven months the Unit was in being, twelve hundred patients were dealt with, the average length of stay in hospital being six to eight weeks. Each block rapidly became a small community with its four wards forming smaller sub-groups; the social structure of these communities followed the pattern of the Effort Syndrome Unit at Mill Hill. Daily talks were held in each block and the mechanisms of psychosomatic symptoms were discussed on two mornings; on the third morning a documentary film was shown followed by a discussion. These films covered such topics as day nurseries, rehabilitation or job training. A fourth morning was devoted to psychodrama followed by a discussion, and the fifth morning to a discussion with the patients about problems affecting the hospital community.

The major sociological development at Dartford occurred in our relations with the local community, the opportunity for such developments being particularly favourable. The war had just ended and public sentiment was very friendly towards the ex-prisoner-of-war; the men were still in uniform and their presence soon became known to the majority of the population of Dartford. Our aim was to try and find social and vocational roles for these patients in the local community while they were still in hospital. This was clearly desirable with patients (provided they were well enough to assume such roles) who had been excluded from normal society for periods of up to five years. Besides speaking at local rotary clubs and the like, I made personal contact with numerous firms, shops and farms. Our problem was explained to them and we ultimately had the active support of over seventy employers. The work available represented a good cross-section of the employments in a small industrial and rural community; the range of choice included farming, dairy farming, market-gardening, building, engineering (both agricultural and general), clerical work, and work in foundries, shipyards, paper mills, chemical factories, printing firms, and numerous small shops. The big factories offered many specialized jobs, e.g. work in electrical maintenance, heating, progress, print room, shipping offices, etc. In this way we built up a potential employment field for our total patient population.

The Government put at our disposal three large buses, which, following separate itineraries, dropped the patients each morning and afternoon at their different occupations, and collected them again two hours later. Naturally some of the patients were too ill to be sent out on what we came to call work therapy, and a carpentry shop was available in hospital for these patients. A nurse was employed full time supervising the attendances at work therapy and acting as liaison between myself and the employers. Patients were allowed to change their occupations as often as they wished. The psychologist came to find this reality testing in actual work-situation more useful than any other form of vocational test.

The degree to which patients actually participated in a work programme naturally varied with the different firms, and the degree of skill or previous training the patient might have. In some cases it amounted to nothing more than a spectator role, and an occasional appeal for help with lifting or some simple routine job; but even under these conditions the patient had an opportunity to become aware of some aspects of the work in question, and more important, to come in contact with the ordinary workmen. The latter were extraordinarily kind and seemed to understand without explanation what was required of them to encourage social participation on the part of the patients. In the big firms the welfare officers gave us enormous help in this sphere. The local employment exchange of the Ministry of Labour gave us every assistance, and we were granted a full-time Disablement Resettlement Officer by the Ministry of Labour; this D.R.O. did splendid work in helping us to find suitable employment in civilian life for our patients on discharge from hospital.

Within the hospital community an active cultural life gradually grew up. Numerous plays were produced and acted before large audiences. These frequently reached a very high standard and were a direct continuation of a dramatic tradition which had grown up in many of the prisoner-of-war camps. Within a few weeks of our initiation a unit newspaper had come into being, called the *Grapevine*, and this continued to be produced weekly during our stay at Dartford. This was the best of the various hospital publications that I personally have seen. It contained a constant fund of humour, was freely illustrated, and did much to relieve tension within the patient community. One famous cover drawing created a sensation and produced repercussions in County Hall (the headquarters of the London County Council and the authority responsible for the hospital administration). It depicted a group of very lean patients pleading with the German prison guard to take them back into the P.o.W. camp, so that they might have a decent square meal. An expert dietician was rapidly dispatched from the local governing body concerned and the food did improve!

We had anticipated considerable trouble over the question of discipline partly from hearsay evidence of ex-prisoner-of-war communities following the First World War, and also because patients cooped up in prison camps for up to five years would naturally be expected to dislike any form of restriction. Here our social development on permissive lines, with free communication between the various groups, prevented serious trouble. The need for some social organization was well known to men who had been in prison camps, and who had in most cases witnessed the disastrous effects of the breakdown of a community structure, and the resulting purely individual struggle for survival. Disciplinary problems were constantly raised in discussion, and guidance from the group sought. The group tended to demand severe punishments for misdemeanours, and clearly sought freedom from anxiety in a community with fairly definite social rules. Contrary to our expectations they demanded a figure of authority, and although free discussion of disciplinary problems was always kept up, any positive action was left to the doctor in charge. The pattern followed in any serious breach of discipline, was to have a friendly talk with the patient explaining the social structure of the unit, and the need to maintain this structure in order to give security to the patient population as a whole. It was explained that there was no personal malice involved, but that if the trouble continued the man would have to be sent to another community; in practice this meant being sent to a certain Army convalescent depot where the psychiatrist was fully informed regarding the case, and no punitive action was taken. Periodically, discharges of this kind did occur, but the method seemed to work well in that, patients seen for a second time knew they would be discharged, accepted the situation as a reasonable one, and displayed little or no hostility.

An attempt was made to test the value of the work done by the Dartford community, and a follow-up study was carried out on 100 of our ex-prisoner-of-war patients. Unfortunately it was impossible, for administrative reasons, to obtain a random sample; the first 100 of the 107 patients who had a London residence were finally chosen for this study. They were visited by a psychiatric social worker from three to five months after discharge; in forty-one cases both patient and relatives were seen, in ten cases patients only, and in forty-nine relatives only. The visits were not by appointment, which accounts for the number of men away when visited. The psychiatric social worker used a standard form drawn up by the psychiatrist as the basis for her inquiries, and this was filled up retrospectively.

In a few cases the relatives were considered to be unreliable informants, though the majority were very helpful. Most relatives appeared to understand the purpose of the visit, and were able to give a good account of the patient's condition. Where the relatives' account seemed to be highly subjective or if they described the patient as no better, or worse, a second visit was made in order to see the man himself, and further treatment as an out-patient was suggested where considered necessary.

The relatives, of course, felt the strain of re-adaptation just as the man had done. Some reacted badly, producing additional stress for the patient, and complaining that he had become quieter, or more difficult to please, or that he ate more than his share of the family rations. Others showed remarkable insight into the repatriate's difficulties, and gave striking accounts of his progress. Two mothers attributed their understanding of their sons' difficulties to the experience they had gained when their prisoner-husbands had returned from the World War 1914-18 in a similar condition.

The general picture as far as symptoms go was as follows:

Completely recovered	22
Improved	66
Unimproved	12
	100

Those listed as completely recovered declared they were perfectly well, as well as they had been before the war. Those unimproved all stated they had got somewhat better during their hospital stay, but had again deteriorated when faced with conditions outside; four of the twelve said they were still better than on admission to hospital, while eight said they were as ill as at any previous time.

The stresses to which these men were subjected upon discharge were studied, though housing and work only will be reported here. Housing was a major cause of trouble in nearly 50 per cent of the cases; thirty-eight men were living in definitely overcrowded conditions, and more were likely to do so when their families became fully reunited. In several instances the patient was living with his wife, parents, a married sister and her children. Six of the thirty-eight admitted to quarrels with the relatives with whom they were compelled to live. Six others, who were not considered actually overcrowded, were unable to get on with relatives or neighbours living in the same house, and were under considerable emotional stress from this source. In few of these cases did there seem any hope of early relief.

The general situation regarding work resettlement was as follows:

Pre-war jobs	34
New jobs in old trade	18
New trade	40
No work done	8
	——
	100

Of those returned to their pre-war jobs, twenty-seven had decided on this course before coming to hospital, some because of the obligation felt after having had their pay made up by firms during their absence, rather than for a particular preference for the work itself. Four others had decided to return after interviewing the D.R.O. in hospital, and one who had left hospital with other plans in mind had returned in response to family pressure. Two had returned only temporarily while waiting for vacancies in Government training schemes, and one of these felt guilty and unhappy in his job as he alleged older employees were being dismissed in order to make room for the return of Service men. In all, twenty-eight of the thirty-four declared they were satisfactorily resettled and happy in their work. It was somewhat difficult to discover just how their present work status compared with their pre-war position, as often the relatives did not know, and, in any case, the men had only been at work for a short period. As far as could be judged, six had improved in status, and one who had abandoned work for health reasons shortly after starting, had deteriorated. Some of those who had improved appeared to be doing extremely well.

The men who had taken new jobs in their old trade were mostly unskilled men who did not qualify for reinstatement owing to the short time spent in their last pre-war job; there were a few who preferred to find new jobs despite the possibility of reinstatement. Eleven of the eighteen said they were content, and five said they were waiting for a chance to improve their status; two had apparently deteriorated.

Of the forty men who had embarked upon a new trade, twenty-one said they were contented in it. A further five were hoping soon to improve their status—they were waiting for licences to open businesses, or for partners to be demobilized, etc.—and two of these were attending technical schools. In addition three were waiting for Government training. The remaining ten were undecided about their jobs, or were discouraged about them; two of these had had to abandon work for health reasons and were attending out-patient clinics.

Of the eight men who had done no work, one had been in hospital with infectious hepatitis, and one was attending an Army Civilian Resettlement Unit. Of the remaining six who presumably had not started for reason of maladjustment of one sort or another, five stated they felt much improved and this statement tallied with the impressions of relatives and investigator. Only one of them came in the group of twelve unimproved; eleven of these unimproved men had at least begun work though some had had to abandon it. Pre-Army work history was assessed as satisfactory or the reverse, the latter being characterized by much unemployment, frequent changes in job, or any down-grading of status. Seventeen of our one hundred men were classified as having had unsatisfactory pre-war histories, but none of the six non-starters were amongst them. All seventeen had returned to work promptly.

Thus of the total group of one hundred, sixty said they were settled and well contented with their work, and a further sixteen were looking forward to bettering their conditions in the near future. On the other hand, six men did not start work at all for reasons of maladjustment, and three abandoned it because of recurrence of their symptoms. This was a very favourable outcome (compare Lewis,[1] 1943), but we were by no means certain it would persist for long beyond the three- to five-month period of our follow-up; a later follow-up was contemplated but never carried out.

The Government training schemes offered a particularly tempting prospect to the repatriated prisoner-of-war, and twenty-four of our one hundred men applied while in hospital for one or other of the trades in which training was offered. However, three months after discharge only one man was in the training he had applied for. Three others had changed their trade and had begun training. Three more were waiting for their first choice, and two had changed their trade and were waiting for their second choice. Fifteen men had given up waiting, twelve of these being men now engaged in other jobs, and three still out of work. The five who still waited for training all showed great keenness to do so, and between them had a high degree of neurotic symptoms, which could largely be attributed to their unsettled state.

The investigator felt that the delay in starting the course was a definite factor retarding the recovery of those men who had opted for it. Still more were likely to abandon the idea, though not all those who said they no longer wanted to train had actually cancelled the course, and some might later have returned to it. During their period of daily visits to the employment exchange, the patients said they had been given no encouragement whatsoever; on the contrary the exchanges usually encouraged the men to abandon the idea of training, or at least to change to some alternative course where the waiting list was shorter.

At the same time the labour market was very favourable to the neurotic, and a temporary job with good pay was easy to obtain. These were mostly arranged through a friend or casual acquaintance, and very many were in the building trade with local contractors, and had the additional advantage of being near to the patient's home, whereas the Government training often took place at a considerable distance from it. In some cases training involved living in hostels, an arrangement peculiarly repugnant to the neurotic repatriate with his special desire for the security and protection of the home.

The majority of these men, according to the Ministry of Labour D.R.O. and the psychiatrist in charge of them, would have proved good material for training. The training scheme must be said to have failed where these men are concerned, and it is likely that their

[1] Lewis, A., *Lancet*, I, 167, 1943.

condition will deteriorate should they become redundant on an over-crowded labour market in the future. It is at least a possibility that many who could have become skilled workers, will instead ultimately become drifters among the permanently unemployed.

A large number of men, thirty, had decided against the plans they had made whilst in hospital. Fifteen of these were those who had been disappointed over their training courses; the others, in spite of advice received at the hospital, had found quite different work once they had come into contact with the labour market outside.

The explanations given were all very similar. 'I had a friend who knew a man . . . a local contractor talked to my father', even 'the wife's boss said he had a good job going'. It was always through direct personal contact that the job was arranged, and it was precisely because of the intimate nature of the arrangement that the men responded so eagerly. In one case the man had already been back at his old job, and was feeling unable to carry on owing to the noise of the engineering shop, when a casual acquaintance stopped him in the street and offered him work as a joiner in his building firm. Carpentry had always been the man's hobby, and the arrangement proved a very successful one; the patient recovered his self-confidence, and was happy and contented when interviewed. The majority of jobs obtained in this way were of an unskilled or semi-skilled nature, and though in some cases the change of plan was definitely of advantage to the patient, in others his ultimate security may have been jeopardized.

Because of the short-term nature of this follow-up, no statement about the effect of residual illness on working capacity is valid. Actually, only eight men of those who returned to work missed over fourteen days during this period, but on discharge from the Army, these men all got two months' leave with pay, and although the majority (fifty-nine) returned to work before this period expired, some had been at work only a month when visited.

We can to some extent check these results in our sample by reference to a follow-up done by the Ministry of Labour. This consisted of a letter sent to the patient's home three and a half months after his discharge from hospital, and we had the returns for the six-month period July to December, 1945, only. During this period 687 patients were discharged, and 610 (90 per cent) were reported as being in work or training, thirty-one not yet in work, and eight unfit for work. Replies were not received from the patients in twenty cases, and from the local employment exchanges in eighteen. It seems, therefore, that our sample at best does not greatly misrepresent the facts as to the entire group.

The response to treatment shown by the patients at Dartford was in general far better than at either Mill Hill or Belmont. Although this group represented the most maladjusted 1 per cent of the hundred thousand repatriates from the European theatre of war, their relatively good response to treatment suggests, that the truly neurotically predisposed in the Army were either not placed in a position where they were likely to be captured, or were unable to survive the rigours of captive life in Germany without dying or becoming so ill as to be repatriated. As it turned out, our problems had been very similar to those met with in the Army Civilian Resettlement Units (which were for the rehabilitation of the not overtly neurotic repatriate), as we discovered at our first meeting with Wilson[1] (1947) and his associates.

The results of the work done at Dartford, and the much larger experience of the Army with their Civilian Resettlement Units, led to a considerable growth of interest in therapeutic communities. The Ministry of Health decided to establish a unit for the treatment and resettlement of chronic unemployed psychiatric casualties at Sutton Emergency Hospital, which later changed its name to Belmont Hospital.

[1]Wilson, A. T. M., Doyle, M., and Kelnar, J., *Lancet*, 1, 735, 1947.

CHAPTER II

THE INDUSTRIAL NEUROSIS UNIT AT BELMONT HOSPITAL

THIS Unit of one hundred beds was established as part of the Neurosis Centre at Belmont Hospital (formerly known as Sutton Emergency Hospital) in April 1947. It had the backing of the Ministries of Health, Labour and Pensions, and its main function was to study the problem of the chronic unemployed neurotic. As was discussed in the Introduction, the Disabled branch of the Ministry of Labour is much concerned with this group, who constitute a large part of the so-called 'hard core' of the unemployed. In medical circles they are equally well known amongst the chronic attenders at various out-patient departments; they are met in every branch of medicine, and although in some cases they may have an obvious physical complaint, this complaint does not adequately explain the degree of personality and social disorganization which is found. Our aim has been

(1) to study a sample of this group and as far as possible understand its clinical characteristics,

(2) to give appropriate psychiatric treatment,

(3) to decide on the most suitable job,

(4) to arrange resettlement, preferably while the patient is still in hospital, and

(5) to test the effect of these procedures by carrying out an adequate follow-up study.

Cases are sent to this hospital from all parts of England, while all employment exchanges and psychiatric out-patient departments in the country have been informed of the existence of the Unit. An application for admission must be accompanied by a full psychiatric report. Provided the case represents a psychiatric problem, and has employment difficulties, he is almost invariably accepted for admission; we do not, however, accept cases which are frankly psychotic. Our population comprises in the main chronic neurotics and character disorders of a kind usually considered unsuitable for treatment by psychotherapy or physical methods. They are difficult to classify and include inadequate and aggressive psychopaths, schizoid personalities, early schizophrenics, various drug addictions, sexual perversions and the chronic forms of psychoneuroses.

All patients are seen on admission by the doctor in charge, and after a short talk referred to one of the Unit psychiatrists. The admission procedure is regarded as important, and when the patient is informed about a vacancy in the Unit, he is given a written description of the organization of it which clearly distinguishes it from the lay concept of a hospital. After having seen the doctor in charge, the new patient is taken around the hospital, shown the workshops, etc., and accompanied to meals on his first day in hospital by a patient who has volunteered for this reception work. New patients all arrive on Mondays (we admit ten patients per week), and are examined by the psychiatrist within twenty-four hours of admission; they see the psychologist as a matter of routine in the first week, and the Disablement Resettlement Officer and Psychiatric Social Worker as soon as the psychiatrist thinks this is indicated.

The staff of the Unit comprises four psychiatrists, one psychologist, two psychiatric social workers, two disablement resettlement officers of the Ministry of Labour, five occupational instructors, one research technician, and a total nursing staff of about twenty. The workshops cover hairdressing, tailoring, plastering, carpentry and bricklaying, each with its own instructor. No attempt is made to train people for a trade; our aim is to have conditions of work which approximate to those of the factory with the men doing semi-skilled or unskilled work. The patients do not make things for themselves, but as far as possible, are engaged on work of social value; for example, they have converted a large room into numerous small offices for the doctors, and improved the amenities around the tennis court by levelling the ground and building an ornamental wall. Most of our patients have very poor work records with long periods of unemployment, and our aim is to get them back to the habit of work; most placements from hospital are in the unskilled field, so that it is important that the work done in hospital should approximate as far as possible to the working conditions they will find outside. We believe that occupational therapy of the diversional type would be unsuitable for our population; art classes, etc., are encouraged in the patients' spare time, but the routine work day of 10 a.m. to 12 a.m. and 2 p.m. to

4 p.m. must be adhered to. A nurse goes around the workshops daily to check the attendances, and it is constantly stressed to the patients that attendance at the workshop is part of their treatment and full co-operation is essential. A small number of patients are found employment in the neighbouring community. To date, over thirty employers in the Sutton district have helped us in this way. Clearly, we must ourselves consider the patient to be fitted for such work before testing him out on the local community. This form of reality testing which was found so useful in the Dartford experiment, cannot be used to any great extent now; our present population is much more ill than were the patients at Dartford, and the Belmont patients lacked the sentimental appeal of the ex-prisoners-of-war. Nevertheless this method still proves very useful with difficult vocational problems. The same applies to the local Government training centre at Waddon; the Ministry of Labour officials there have been extremely helpful and taken many of our patients for two hours a day, for a trial period, in order to test out their suitability for later full training when they leave hospital.

The patient's occupation while in hospital depends mainly on the patient's own preference, provided this does not run counter to the opinion of the psychologist, the D.R.O., and the patient's own doctor. In such a case the final decision must be worked out between the patient and his psychiatrist. The question of vocational guidance is gone into at length in Chapter IX. We have found tests of aptitude to be of relatively little value; much more important is the man's attitude towards work, and to tasks in general, whether they be vocational, social or recreational. This problem is discussed further in Chapter VIII.

A placement conference is held weekly, and attended by all members of the staff of the Unit. The doctor in charge of the case reads out a brief statement of the problem, mainly from the employment angle, although of course the medical factors must also be considered. Separate reports are then read out expressing the opinions of the other members of the resettlement team. The psychologist reports on the man's intelligence (Mill Hill Vocabulary and Progressive Matrices tests, and Wechsler I.Q.), results of the vocational tests, if these have been used, and any additional tests, for example, projection and deterioration tests. In addition to this information, the psychologist is able to report on the patient's behaviour during the tests, his assessment of the results and his final opinion regarding job placement. The D.R.O. reports on the man's previous work record, his present work interests, and the opportunities for such work in the man's home area; at this stage the man may have already been sent for interview to several prospective employers. In any case the D.R.O. will have seen the man on numerous occasions, had consultation with the other members of the resettlement team, and will usually have come to a fairly definite opinion as to the man's employment prospects. The occupational instructor or outside employer furnishes a report regarding the man's behaviour during working hours, his interest, his social adjustment, adaptability, persistence, and any skills he may have demonstrated. The ward nurse reports on the man's adjustment to the other patients and to herself, his behaviour at meals, attitude towards the ward fatigues and leisure activities. Finally, the Psychiatric Social Worker may have been in contact with the man to discuss any domestic problems, and may have done a home visit; her information about home circumstances and so on may help in determining the type of accommodation, etc., required. The doctor in charge of the case summarizes the information contained in these various reports, in the form of a digest, which includes the final opinion arrived at by the placement conference after due discussion. A copy of this digest is sent to the man's local employment exchange on his discharge from hospital. A conference of this type integrates the whole work of the Unit and exerts a steady educational influence on the individual staff members. The patient himself is interviewed by the conference when this is considered necessary.

Approximately a third of our patients are considered to be unemployable in the open labour market. Except in the case of frank psychotics, etc., such a decision is seldom arrived at before a trial period of six to eight weeks in hospital; even then we frequently defer decision, hoping that a further month or two in the therapeutic environment of the Unit, may bring about sufficient clinical and social improvement to justify an attempt at job placement. We normally have visitors from various social science fields and from many different countries sitting in at these conferences; much useful criticism has been offered by them. In this placement conference, probably the greatest weakness is the absence of direct contact with the employment field. This could be met more readily if we were serving the local community, but out-patients come from all over the country. The Regional Technical Adviser from the Ministry of

Labour, J. Sprackling, gives us valuable assistance on practical problems relating to working conditions and the employment field generally, but even his presence does not altogether compensate for the absence of any doctor with first-hand experience in the industrial field.

The patients' day follows a definite pattern; breakfast is over by 8 a.m. and from then until 9 a.m. the patients do their fatigues designed to keep the ward tidy. Every week morning from 9 a.m. to 10 a.m. there is some form of community meeting attended by all the patients on the Unit, the nurses who can be spared, and any of the other Unit staff who can afford the time. The purpose of these meetings is discussed in Chapter IV under Social Therapies. Briefly, on Monday there is a Unit conference when the patients air their grievances or make constructive suggestions. Problems raised are discussed fully, and we aim at solutions agreeable to the majority. The doctor in charge invariably takes this meeting since whenever possible final decisions are made without delay; we have found it important to work through a problem at the time it is raised, otherwise it is liable to arouse anxiety or lead to the growth of rumour. On Tuesdays, films dealing with job training, social problems, rehabilitation, etc., are shown on a sound projector. Wednesdays and Thursdays are devoted to a discussion group taken by one of the Unit staff, and on Fridays a psychodrama is presented. From 10 a.m. to 12 noon and from 2 p.m. to 4 p.m. patients are at their occupations as already described; from 4 p.m. to 7 p.m., if well enough to be granted a pass, the patients may leave the hospital grounds. From 7 p.m. until bedtime, at 9 p.m., they have an organized social programme prepared by a committee elected from among the patients, this is readily censured at the group discussions should it fail to cater for all needs. In addition to the usual socials, whist drives, concerts, dances, etc., there are beginners' dancing classes, play reading groups, and an art class; indeed any creative activity is encouraged. Ample facilities exist for such games as cricket, football, tennis, badminton, etc. These social activities are constantly referred to as part of the treatment; the nurses actively participate, taking care to encourage the more backward and inhibited patients, and avoiding the temptation of 'seduction' by the more attractive ones.

The average length of stay in hospital is from two to four months; a certain number stay for considerably longer periods of up to a year; others stay a much shorter time and some even leave of their own accord within a few hours of arrival in hospital.

Each psychiatrist carries a case load of twenty to thirty patients and has two or three admissions per week. Individual treatment is mainly on supportive lines, and relatively few patients receive uncovering types of therapy. A small number of patients have received from twenty to one hundred hours of psychotherapy; none have received psychoanalytic treatment. Facilities exist for all known physical methods of psychiatric treatment. Modified insulin treatment is used extensively, and there are always a few patients on electrical convulsive therapy. Abreactive techniques with ether or sodium amytal are used very occasionally, as is the operation of leucotomy. Insulin coma treatment is used fairly frequently, but continuous narcosis hardly at all.

This hospital is run by the Ministry of Health so all treatment is free. Many of the patients are in receipt of war pensions, and during their stay in hospital the Ministry of Pensions gives them an allowance of eleven shillings per week pocket money; some of the patients have considerably less than this to spend. The social workers have to meet constant demands for clothing as many of the patients are literally threadbare. A prolonged stay in hospital frequently means severe financial hardship for the patient's family.

Belmont Hospital itself, of which the Unit is a part, is a drab building originally built as a workhouse. There is a minimum of physical comfort but the canteen facilities are good, and the recreation rooms large and cheerful. The grounds are quite the pleasantest part of the hospital environment.

CHAPTER III

THE SOCIAL STRUCTURE OF THE INDUSTRIAL UNIT

STAFF

IN order to understand the structure of our staff community, we must first study and clarify the roles of the various categories constituting the group. A role is a set of legitimate expectations of behaviour, and the cohesiveness of any social structure depends on the effectiveness of the performance of important roles. We want to conceptualize our ideas regarding the various roles in our hospital community, but are fully aware that there will frequently be considerable discrepancy between our conception of a role and the individual's actual performance; this is particularly true in the case of the patient role.

Nurses

The nurses are numerically the largest group and in many ways the most important. As has already been explained, the majority of our nurses have had no previous nursing training either as general or mental nurses. We have a small nucleus of trained nurses to deal with our physically ill patients and supervise the physical methods of treatment. Apart from them, we have in the main, girls who are aiming to do some form of social work and who have preferably got a university degree in one of the social sciences. Such people cannot be expected to work for long at an assistant nurse's rate of pay (£8 per month with full board), but we get a steady stream of this type of girl who comes for six months to a year in order to get practical experience in psychiatry and sociology. Many of our nurses come from Scandinavia and particularly from Norway. The fact that they are foreigners seems to have certain advantages. Our de-socialized patients feel themselves to be outside the community and in this sense are also 'foreigners'; frequently they seem to accept the foreign nurse with greater readiness than they do the Britisher. However, it is probable that the new British nurse is in a similar relationship with the patient; her feelings of strangeness are felt by the patients and tend to arouse the desire to help her fit into the community. Almost imperceptibly she comes to take on her more permanent role of friend and sympathizer, herself offering the security and stability so needed in our community. Yet even in the earliest days the nurse will appreciate the differences of personalities and needs among the patients; many will readily offer 'protective' advice and encouragement, while others will at first be apprehensive of the intruder and her possible challenge to the *status quo*.

There is no preliminary training school for the nurses of the Industrial Unit, and they start work immediately on the wards. As already described, they have a daily tutorial from a psychiatrist, but the initiation is mainly through another nurse on the same ward. If this nurse is a person with a well-developed social sense and a clear idea of the aims of the Unit, then the traditions will be imparted readily, as at this initial period possible hostile reactions in the new nurse will be strongly inhibited, while there will be a relatively great capacity and need for imitation. The anti-social nurse/instructor will, of course, have an equally favourable opportunity to 'infect' the new nurse with her dissatisfaction during the induction period, but if the nursing traditions are well established there will be no serious threat to the group structure. The problems facing the new nurse are brought out in the following extract from a nurse's paper on the role of the nurse. At the weekly staff meeting everyone takes it in turn to write a paper on their place in the Unit team; this paper was read by a nurse four weeks after her arrival in the Unit, when the difficulties of the induction period were fresh in her mind.

'During the first few days, when it was quite impossible to think about anything but how to find one's way about and how to get into the routine of the duties, one impression forced itself upon me. This was that the Unit was an exceptionally nice place to work in because of the friendliness of the atmosphere. This friendliness was extended to me from doctors, nurses and patients, and it took very little time for me to feel at ease, though not necessarily having much understanding. I think this is immensely important—that ease in the assimilation of a new nurse should take precedence over any technical training. I kept a rough diary for the first few weeks and I find comments about the pleasantness of the atmosphere recurring constantly. The same thing was noticeable in the wards—the patients did far more for me in the first few days than I could hope to do for them.

'Apart from personal relationships, the atmosphere was particularly congenial as it was plain from the first that any expected pattern of behaviour is not that of a ward orderly emptying ashtrays and folding counterpanes, but a nurse who does these routine duties carefully, realizing their necessity in maintaining some standards of cleanliness and tidiness, and then gives all her intelligence to understanding and helping with the social research function of the Unit. The daily nurses' tutorials, this staff meeting, and so on, all reinforce the feeling that the Unit is a research team, aiming at finding out more about neurosis, and more important from my point of view, about the mechanisms of social life. We are expected to understand our own part in the structure of this community and help to make that structure an integrated one; we want the Unit to be the best possible place for people who have become maladjusted to their society, to become more socialized. Of course, this is an ambitious aim, and it is for that reason that the constant discussion of the Unit social structure is so important.

'These then were my first impressions—the friendliness and stimulation of the atmosphere. For the first two weeks I was immensely excited by new experiences and learning new things. However, my mood passed to one of bewilderment and some unhappiness. Yes, this was a fine place and the work was fascinating, but here are all these people, unhappy and worried, and what on earth could I do about it? I think these feelings of inadequacy are bound to come because it is part of the role of the nurse to receive some of the patients' own bitterness, resentment and hostility. However, this concept doesn't help the new nurse to cope with her own emotions at the time, because in all probability she is unprepared for them. For this reason, because the emotional content of the work is so great, I feel that a new nurse should be helped towards a little insight at the beginning. Of course I don't know how typical my own reaction is —so this is purely tentative. Dr. Maxwell Jones has, I know, the idea of writing a guide for the new nurse, and this presumably would embody some such instruction. As the weeks have gone on, I myself have become much more aware of my own role, and I now know these feelings of inadequacy are shared by everyone in the Unit.

'My own conception of the role of the nurse at the moment is largely second-hand, because I have not had time to do any reconstruction even if that is necessary. One of the things I feel is most vital is that the nurse-patient role should be made very clear, so that the patient recognizes a common pattern of behaviour in all the nursing staff. I have written here a short and incomplete summary of my conception of this role.

'First, the nurse must display a well-adjusted personality. She must avoid being either too serious or too flippant—to encourage the weak senses of humour of her patients—to act as a sympathizer but as a stimulator too. She must be cheerful, laugh and chat and dance and be interested all the time. For this reason it is important that there shall be plenty of nurses, because though the ward and cafeteria work doesn't amount to very much, when one is looking after one ward alone it is nearly impossible to have much time left over for individual chatting. I think the patients miss this when pressure of work deprives them of it.

'Secondly, the more complex role of the nurse is to be the receiver of patients' hostility, aggression and so on, and not be unduly depressed or worried by it. In conjunction with this patient-nurse relationship there goes the doctor-nurse one—the nurse must try and understand case papers, not so that she can act in a therapeutic capacity but so that she can try to understand what the patient is doing in his relationship to her.

'Thirdly, swinging away from the patient-nurse relationship, the nurse's role in this Unit is to understand and help to strengthen the total social structure as I have said before.

'How far any particular nurse fills her role will depend largely on her own personality and intelligence. In this work it is essential that a good deal of spontaneity is preserved, and that the nurses should be free, when they have completed their official duties, to use their interest in the most constructive way possible for them.'

Another new nurse wrote six weeks after her arrival on the Unit. . . .

'What indications does the new nurse receive as to her expected behaviour? On arriving she will have some vague idea of the way the Unit is run, and information of a general kind will be passed on by the previous generation of nurses, or from the published description of the Unit, or gleaned at the daily tutorials. But the most important side will come from the patients themselves; at first glance there is nothing wrong with them, so obviously it is not the "Nightingale" touch which is required, a point which was made clear to me on my first day when an embarrassed-looking man tapped me on the shoulder, and indicating another patient who practically cowered, said, "Excuse me nurse, there's a man here wants to change his trousers." Evidently we have no aura of blanket baths and bedpan.

'Since then I have heard a patient say that he regarded the staff nurses as the equivalent of the Army medical orderlies, and the female assistants as social workers; another was more succinct—we were Gestapo. It is suggested that we are unconsciously mother-images, therefore as members of the staff of the hospital we are representatives of authority who must at times enforce rules. In our more social duties we are friends and encouragers, and in our dual capacity there are twin dangers to beware of; first, that we may usurp or accept authority, giving orders instead of encouragement, and making decisions for people who should make their own, or having one's words treated as oracular pronouncements; and second, the risk of demotion, for there is constant tendency to render the nurse harmless by trapping her into a new false position, by seeking physical contact or by enlisting ready sympathies on their side against the world, and forcing acceptance of their unreal standards. The man who told me that I was not "cut out for this sort of work" was seeking to immobilize me rather than making a serious con-tribution to my employment problems. There was probably a similar motive behind the request by one member of the group on Monday morning to have the staff put on their psychodramas.

'Our uniform and title play a considerable part, I imagine, in help-ing us to walk our tight rope, making it quite plain that we are not just friendly women who happen to be around the place; we may not be "proper" nurses, but we share something of the respect due to the stripy cloth.'

Let us now consider the nurse/patient relationship as this is the biggest single problem facing the nurse. What is her role in relation to the patient? If this is left undefined, then the patient or group of patients have every incentive to project whatever anti-social or other feelings they wish, on to the person of the nurse. She can, if she is identified with authority, be the doctor's stooge or mistress, a spy, or a two-faced liar, or if simply seen as a woman, may be desirable or feared, according to the psycho-sexual make-up or mood of the individual. If we continue to think of the nurse in this featureless role, she will probably not intervene when trouble arises in the ward, as for example a quarrel between two patients one of whom is supporting the ward ruling regarding lights out at 10 p.m. This may well be interpreted by the defaulting patient as approval or even encouragement of his anti-social behaviour, and may arouse tensions in the entire group who need to feel that there is a positive group structure and discipline to guide them, of which the nurse is a representative. But the nurse must be identified with both authority and the patient group, and of course her position is made much more pleasant if these two groups themselves are clearly defined, and in close contact with each other.

It is convenient to consider the nurse's role under three general headings—authoritarian, social and therapeutic. What about her authoritarian role? The nurse will find her response to problems presented by the patients (such as an attempt to involve her in a quarrel among themselves) gradually changing. At first she may act almost intuitively; later she may find that her concern to act appropriately almost inhibits a confident and ready response; ultimately as her experience widens she will find that she has largely assimilated the trends of the community and has a deeper understanding of the motives behind the patients' behaviour. Should the nurse take positive action when some ward rule or cultural pattern is violated? In general we have tried to avoid this and simply ask the nurse to report such matters, which are then dealt with by the doctor in charge working in close collaboration with the sister. It might be argued that this is viewed by the patients as a combination of hostility and weakness on the part of the nurse. I think this can be overcome by a clear awareness by the patients of the group structure as a whole—it emphasizes the need for a positive pattern, clearly understood not only by the staff, but by the patients as well. In fact the main problem confronting us at present is how to clarify our different staff roles, and, having done so, how to work as harmoniously as possible as an integrated whole. But along with this, at every stage, is the imperative necessity to convey to the patients an awareness of this structure so that it is as well known to them as to ourselves. To return to the nurses' disciplinary role, I think they must align themselves with 'authority', and interfere actively in extreme cases—e.g.—two patients fighting. In less severe infractions—e.g. a patient absenting himself from his occupation—they must report the incident leaving it to be dealt with by the doctor in charge. In minor infractions—e.g. throwing cigarette ends on the ward floor—they should indicate their opinion that the 'official' view is a reasonable one but are not required to take any other positive action. The nurse should realize that the patient community needs a positive discipline in order to protect it from its more anti-social elements, so that in carrying out her authoritarian role she is meeting a community need.

The social role of the nurse is an all important one, and for this reason our 'nurses' would be more aptly termed 'social workers'. She must attempt to understand the patients' individual problems; in this she is helped by reading the case notes, and by the daily tutorials. Each nurse has approximately seventeen patients to look after, but unfortunately each ward contains twice this number of men, and she cannot ignore the remaining half; this makes it much more difficult for the individual nurse to have her patients as an integrated group. She cannot spend an equal amount of time with each of her patients, but must distribute her time according to circumstances and the needs of her patients. Thus the demanding hysteric, whose craving for affection can never be satisfied, might attempt to appropriate her largely for himself; whereas the disgruntled man in the corner bed who refuses to participate in any of the group activities, may be more helped by her attention, even though he snubs her and asks to be left alone.

The nurse must constantly guard against satisfying her own needs rather than ministering to the patients'; the temptation is to spend time with those patients who make her feel welcome and whose company she enjoys. She must be prepared to be flexible and not adhere to any one social formula; there will always be some social patients who cannot, or do not want to participate in group activities—these patients' desires should be respected and their individual needs considered just as much as the more 'social' needs of the average patient. Periodically throughout her working day the nurse should ask herself what each of her patients is doing, and if uncertain, take steps to find out. Thus, if during a ward social she realizes that all but two of her patients are present she should satisfy herself that the two absent members are not feeling rejected or overlooked. She must be prepared to take the initiative at a dance, and if she considers it necessary ask an inhibited patient to dance. In this social role she is not behaving as a woman but as a social worker; she is not be-having according to *her* sexual and social needs but attempting to give her patients a feeling of security and of being understood. The sexual factor is inevitably present, just as it is between parents and child, but it must be sacrificed to the greater need of the neurotic patient for an understanding parent figure. The integrity of the nurses' group can be upset by the indiscretion of any one member; a nurse who allows her sexual needs to be met in an overt way by the patients will alter the patients' attitude towards the whole nursing group, and make the nurses' therapeutic role a less effective one. Although the patients constantly try to make 'dates' with the nurses, they do not really want them as sexual objects as much as they need them as non-sexual parent figures; they can find sexual partners almost anywhere, and much of the value of the nurse to them lies in the very fact that they can have a relationship with an understand-ing woman without the anxieties associated with a sexual affair. It must be remembered that practically every neurotic has severe problems and anxieties of a sexual nature, and apart altogether from the nursing role, a girl would be ill advised to become involved in such conflicts.

Finally, let us consider the treatment role of the nurse. In general one may say that the nurse does not participate in a psychothera-peutic relationship with any one patient. Her role is more to interpret or transmit the Unit culture to the patient; the more she has accepted this culture, the more readily and competently can she fulfil her role. She will thus aim not only to encourage and support the patient when his condition calls for this, but she will also attempt to get him to participate in the various social, work, and community treatment activities such as psychodrama. When the patient grumbles about the necessity to go to his work therapy or to the daily discussion groups, the nurse will give a consistent interpretation of the Unit culture in respect of these two activities and encourage him to raise his grievance in the discussion group.

The nurse will frequently be sought out by the patients and asked questions which may appear to force her into a semi-therapeutic role. As a general principle I feel that the nurse need not refuse to be drawn into discussions which touch on patients' neurotic problems, but she must limit herself to a purely 'supportive' or encouraging role and not attempt any interpretations. She may be able to make some tentative suggestions but in general she will refer the patient back to his doctor. It may be that in certain special instances a more active therapeutic role may be played by the nurses acting in close collaboration with the doctor—e.g. as a member of a small therapeutic group, or as the producer of a psychodrama. But in general the nurse's treatment activity is limited to her transmission of the Unit culture to the patients and any specific role which she may be given to play by the doctor at the daily nurses' tutorial. Thus she may be asked to be particularly passive and indulgent with a man whose control over his aggression is almost gone, while at a later date it may be expedient to treat the same patient in a much more active way.

In conclusion, the nurse must be constantly on the look-out for emotional involvements with patients, and realize that more often than not these are the form of 'acting out' on the part of a patient, and do not refer to her personally but rather to her as a substitute for someone else; thus a patient, whose treatment interviews with the doctor has made conscious or near conscious latent hostility towards his mother may displace this hostility on to any convenient person in his immediate environment—probably the nurse. In the same way the nurse must guard against being roused to anger, etc., by accounts of neglect and maltreatment from the patient's doctor, where the origin of hostility may well refer to a deep-seated hatred dating from early childhood which is being aroused in the treatment situation. It is for this and other reasons that it might be argued that ideally every nurse on the Unit should have been psychoanalysed; this is clearly impracticable even if desirable, but much can be done in the daily nurses' tutorials to make the nurses aware of transference phenomena. This point is developed in detail in Dr. Freeman's chapter on 'Some Problems of In-Patient Psychotherapy'. The doctor may be greatly helped in his treatment of a case by the nurses' reports of these extra analytic transference situations.

We have described a very simple concept of the role of the nurse. Were our nurses to stay for periods longer than six to twelve months, the role would undoubtedly become much more complex.

Doctors

In our culture the role of the doctor is still associated with a certain amount of magic and is nearer to that of the witchdoctor than many people realize. There seems little doubt that much of the magic associated with medicine has been carried over to the lay concept of the psychiatrist, and the steady stream of films and books on psychiatric topics with which the public is fed has probably contributed largely to this state of affairs. In our chronic neurotic population, however, many of the patients have drifted from doctor to doctor and from hospital to hospital; in the process much of the magic may have been lost and may well have been replaced by resistance to doctors in general and psychiatrists in particular.

In most psychiatric hospitals the doctor behaves towards the patients and nurses much as he would in a general hospital, except in relation to the psychiatric interview itself. Nor is the patient aware of any fundamental difference between a physician and a psychiatrist; certainly he is just as much 'Doctor' as—say—a surgeon or gynaecologist. In the Unit we have attempted to develop the role of the doctor to meet our own limited treatment goal and have tried to avoid pretence. This has meant a considerable break from hospital tradition. We do not dress to conform to the usual concept of the professional man. We have all avoided the white coat, prominent stethoscope, and aggressive percussion hammer as extensions of our body image. The relationship to the patients is a complex one and one which we do not fully understand ourselves. Certainly it is far removed from that of the analyst and at the other extreme we are by no means absorbed into the patient community. The patients' attitude towards the doctor is usually an ambivalent one. He is a miracle worker who should be able to solve all their problems; but he is also a figure of authority who may be feared and distrusted. We aim to modify these attitudes and bring the role of the doctor into a much more realistic perspective. The doctor's role in relation to the patients may be considered in five main aspects—social, supportive, by example, activating and interpretive.

The tendency is for the doctors to participate fairly freely in social situations and at social functions. Meeting patients informally or talking and dancing with them at Unit socials are common. Visits to the wards and workshops are also usual. This role is continued after the patient leaves hospital particularly if he chooses to attend the Ex-Patient Club which meets weekly in the centre of London. The adoption of such a social role usually modifies the patient's concept of the doctor in the direction of a more benign authority.

The supportive role of the doctor is linked with his social role but goes further. In various treatment situations where no interpretive approach is possible or desirable the doctor (like the nurse) is helping the patient in every possible way to attain some realistic goal. Thus appreciation of work in the workshops, of progress in the dancing class, or of striving to enact a psychodrama, all call for the doctor's support, and to the patients become part of his familiar role. In this protective setting the patient is given the maximum encouragement to participate in the Unit's therapeutically orientated activities.

The daily discussion group with the entire patient population affords an excellent opportunity for education or modification of behaviour by example. At almost every such meeting hostility is expressed towards the doctor. This may be met by some explanation or even interpretation or be accepted without comment. There are no reprisals or show of anger. Daily occurrences of this kind including all the doctors are one instance of teaching by example and are important in the development of the Unit culture.

Probably more important is the need to stimulate the patient to play an active role. If we consider a Unit discussion group where a patient or group of patients complain to the doctor taking the meeting that they are receiving no treatment and that nothing is being done to help them. One patient may say that he feels no better than when he first came to hospital; he is terribly worried because his wife is in a T.B. sanatorium and his children are being neglected by his sister-in-law who is looking after them. The doctor may reply that the wife is presumably being given the best available treatment for her T.B. but that she is probably at least equally worried about the children; in addition she has the worry about her husband's ill-ness and his inability to be with the children at such an important time. The doctor may initiate a sociodrama where the patient pays a visit to his sister-in-law (played by another patient or nurse). In this acting out or verbal discussion the aim is to get the patient to play an active role or at least test out the possibility of change. The skill with which various doctors can induce this activity in patients varies considerably as do the techniques which they employ. The fact remains that it is one of the most important roles that the doctors are called on to play. This type of active participation can also be achieved in a small therapeutic group (Jones, 1948).[1]

Interpretation in the large discussion groups or in psychodrama is possible to only a very limited extent but can, of course, be used much more readily in the small therapeutic groups and in individual treatment. These aspects of the role of the doctor are discussed in Chapters IV, V and VI.

[1] Jones, M., *Brit. J. Med. Psychol.*, 21, 104, 1948.

The administration of such discipline as is considered necessary is left entirely to the doctor in charge. Defaulters reported by the nurses are seen each morning by the senior doctor and nurse. The situation is discussed and some attempt made to understand the motive behind the misdemeanour. If the patient is too ill to be responsible for his behaviour the matter is regarded as a symptom, and the problem is referred to the doctor concerned. If, on the other hand, the defaulter is considered to be well enough to be responsible, an attempt is made to explain to him the need for any society to establish its own standards of behaviour; these needs have been discussed on frequent occasions in the discussion groups, where the patients clearly demonstrated their need for a disciplinary authority as a means of protection for them against known and hidden dangers. In this sense the defaulters have gone against the culture of the group, and we try to explain to them the need for some discipline in order to preserve the existing group structure. If, following such an explanation, a defaulter persists in his anti-social behaviour, then the question of discharge from the Unit may have to be raised. This is never done without discussion with the doctor concerned, and there must be an adequate disposal available so that the man's mental health is not adversely affected. Inevitably the problem becomes known to the patient body who raise it at one of the daily discussion groups. In actual fact we have had one or two such discharges each year, and we have come to accept the fact that there are certain psychiatric cases (mostly severe character disorders) which cannot be absorbed by our therapeutic community as it is at present constituted.

Finally, the doctor–nurse relationship needs to be considered. The nurses live in the hospital and come into frequent contact with the doctors in ordinary social activities such as mealtimes. The staff eat in a large cafeteria with separate tables. In addition to the Unit staff the entire hospital use this cafeteria. The hospital doctors tend to eat together, apart from their nurses, whereas the Unit doctors, nurses, etc., tend to be drawn together. Surnames are used more commonly than christian names, but this varies from time to time and is accentuated by an influx of new nurses. The tendency is for the doctors to use the nurses' christian names and for the nurses to retain the title 'doctor' particularly if anyone from outside the Unit is present. The relationship between nurses and doctors is under constant review at the staff meetings and often results in considerable tension. This has applied in particular to matters bearing on the traditional (hospital) relationship between the sister (charge nurse) and the other nurses. Considerable anxiety and jealousy has at times been felt as a result of what has been interpreted by the sister as the doctor's intrusion into the nursing sphere. Difficulties of this kind are inevitable in view of the wide differences between the Unit culture and the established traditions of nursing. However, we have been lucky in having had two sisters during the life of the Unit, both of whom were able to adjust to the new traditions.

Daily contact with the nurses in tutorials, etc., and the whole social structure of the Unit make for an unusually good understanding between nurses and doctors. The fact that most nurses have not had a nursing training, that some have had training in the social science fields, that the majority come from foreign countries and that all have applied to work on the Unit as a result of a particular interest in this type of work, has considerably simplified the establishment of a good nurse-doctor relationship.

Disablement Resettlement Officers (D.R.O.s)

This account of the role of the D.R.O. in the Unit has been written by Miss Elizabeth Cann, one of our two full-time D.R.O.s seconded to the Unit by the Ministry of Labour.

'The role of a D.R.O. in a therapeutic community is a much easier one than the same role in an employment exchange. The physical fact that the D.R.O.s are employed full-time on the Unit premises and not in the employment exchange favourably affects the attitude of the patient to the D.R.O. and vice versa. There is no waiting public to increase the patient's anxiety and to antagonize him before he sees the D.R.O., and the interview can be conducted in an atmosphere which is not clouded by reference to medical reports, registration as a disabled person, and eligibility for unemployment benefit. The D.R.O. becomes known to the patient as someone whom he sees frequently chatting in the wards, attending group meetings, contributing to discussions, showing films on types of job, rehabilitation or social problems, and giving talks on the Disabled Persons (Employment) Act, training courses and other Ministry of Labour activities. To a demanding neurotic this attention means a great deal. He is pleased, slightly flattered maybe, and frequently accepts the fact that a serious attempt is being made to tackle his employment problem. It is this positive attitude towards the D.R.O. which is all important if a successful outcome is to ensue.

'The advantages acquired through the ability to shed official atmosphere and approach in this way cannot be over-emphasized, but this of itself is of little avail unless supported by the internal structure of the Unit. Through this the D.R.O. is enabled to study the patient as a whole human being. His case history recreates his background and makes clear any environmental stresses and emotional difficulties; his behaviour in the ward, in the social life of the Unit, in the morning community group, and in the workshop, is an invaluable guide to the man's present capacity to adjust to the various stresses he may meet either socially or at work. All this can be observed at first-hand by the D.R.O. Discussion with the psychiatrist makes clear to what extent the man's stay in the Unit is likely to improve his ability to cope with his particular difficulties and gives much needed guidance as to the degree of limitation imposed on a patient with high-grade intelligence because of his poor personality. Discussion of the man's behaviour and ability with the nurse and workshop instructor with whom he spends most of the day is a very real practical supplement to the psychologist's assessment of the man's intelligence, personality and aptitude. All these collected facts and impressions are watched and studied by the D.R.O. as the man's psychiatric treatment proceeds. With this fore-knowledge of each other the first hurdle is over. Except in a minority of cases the patient accepts the D.R.O. as a practical member of the therapeutic team, and the D.R.O. has acquired the confidence in handling him which is the natural outcome of the knowledge gained by a study of his whole personality.

'When the stage in a man's treatment is reached for the discussion of a work goal, the method of approach to this topic is of some importance. A casual chat in the workshop, ward or hospital grounds about jobs in general has often led to a good D.R.O.-patient relationship. The reverse would most certainly have been the case with some patients if the normal practice was used of including them in a list of names with interview times. Under these circumstances some might not have come for interview at all, others might have come unwillingly and suspiciously, having seen in the arrangement a possible rejection by the psychiatrist and the approach of their discharge from hospital; this would mean strengthening their resistance to finding employment and so leaving the shelter and security of the hospital. Many patients have no interest in working and no idea whatever as to the type of work they wish to do or are likely to obtain. With this type of case it is necessary to do much inquiry into work possibilities and impossibilities, and to arouse interest and foster ideas by every possible means. If a neurotic has an idea that he can do a certain type of work it is not enough just to tell him that it is not a reasonable suggestion, he requires proof of this. Unless these ideas are thoroughly explored, it is hopeless to try and effect any sort of compromise between the man's demands and the limitations of the labour market for neurotics.

'The demands are mainly for a secure job, e.g. with the Government or local government; a position of trust or authority, e.g. caretaker, park-keeper, policeman; social work, e.g. nursing, welfare officer, D.R.O. "I could easily do your job if I was given a chance" or "People often come to see me for advice and say that I have helped them", are remarks often made by these enthusiasts. Other demands include a job with prospects, and these have to be pretty obvious; a job offering accommodation in the case of men with inadequately housed families; e.g. a farm job with a cottage; a Government training course—"I have never had a trade".

'At the other end of the scale are the restless psychopaths who want to get away from England, to go whale fishing, deep-sea diving, to join the Merchant Navy. Some few would be content just to do a job that keeps them continually on the move—e.g. lorry driving.

'All these would be reasonable demands from fit men, but with the exception of Government courses they are practically all in the pipe-dream class for members of the Unit population. Very rarely a miracle does occur and the need is met, but as a general rule considerable modification is required. Without the psychiatrist's support at this stage the D.R.O. would have an almost hopeless task in giving the man what he would consider to be an adequate substitute work-goal; together they can try to effect a gradual change in the man's attitude to the suggested alternative. Quite often these attempts are treated with scorn until the time for discharge is reached, when there may be last minute capitulation.

'Applications for Government training courses from Unit patients have been accorded priority of allocation, and are in consequence relatively easy to obtain. Thus the temptation to have recourse to them is not easily resisted. Patients frequently regard a training course as the answer to all their difficulties and it is very hard to convince those who clearly are unsuitable subjects that vocational training would serve no useful purpose in their cases.

'In the search for jobs the difficulties have to be experienced to be believed. Our patient population is drawn from the entire country. This means that in most cases the D.R.O.s have no direct contact with the employment position in the region in which the patient is to be employed. The establishment of a good contact with someone in the areas which supply the majority of our patients is of vital importance. The unique knowledge of local employment conditions possessed by local D.R.O.s enables them to assess the opportunities for employment for any particular patient. Often however, a local D.R.O. is restricted in his endeavours to find a job for a Unit patient because of the high proportion of unemployed disabled persons on his register who suffer from neurosis in some form or other, and because of the relatively few suitable opportunities for placing unemployed persons handicapped in this way. Recourse has then to be made to other sources of information, such as trade union officials trade associations and chambers of trade. Patients themselves may frequently be able to supply names of firms who may be interested and, of course, trade journals and the General Post Office classified trade directory are invaluable aids.

'Employers generally have displayed willingness to consider employment possibilities for patients and a genuine desire to help. If wanting the type of labour offered, they will interview the patient; if not they will frequently supply information as to the state of the labour market and how the patient is likely to fare elsewhere. In recommending a patient to an employer emphasis is laid on the points which seem to be of value to the employer. This requires ingenuity at times, but after approaching four or more employers it is surprising how adept one can become. The best employers want to know as much as possible about the prospective employee. Some patients do not wish their stay in hospital to be disclosed; if an explanation of the man's illness is called for it is sometimes more readily understood if it can be related to war experiences, domestic anxiety, unsuitable work, etc.

'Often the employer needs as much, if not more, reassurance regarding the patient's possible conduct, as the patient does regarding his suitability for the work. When job interviews are arranged by the Unit D.R.O.s the patient is given every possible information about the working conditions and a timed appointment is made with the employer. A patient's unwillingness to go for an interview may show itself in many ways. He may refuse the type of work, to work in the area suggested, or under the existing conditions. He may produce reasons which prevent him from going for interview—e.g. losing his glasses, having a "bilious attack", falling down stairs, injuring arms or legs in games; or he may behave at the interview in such a way as to cause the employer to decide not to engage him. Having reached the stage when the patient is prepared to consider the employment found for him he must if possible be shielded from further setbacks. The frustration caused by being turned down at an interview is often enough to result in a considerable loss of confidence, and it may take weeks to bring the patient again to the point when he can contemplate further employment.

'The support and assistance given by the Ministry of Labour District Technical Officer both in assessing a patient's value on the current labour market, and in making direct contacts with understanding employers, has been of immeasurable value to the D.R.O.s. The Technical Officer attends the weekly placement conference at the Unit. His knowledge of the employers' needs, and the standard of worker required, enables him to advise about the likelihood of obtaining the employment desired by the patient, or recommended by the conference. Like the patients, the psychiatrists, psychologists and D.R.O.s are often tempted to aim for jobs a little higher than industry can provide, and the inclusion in the conference of a member able to keep its aims at a reality level has been invaluable. Frequently, when visiting employers, he has interested them in the work of the Unit, and has effected very satisfactory placements for patients.

'The question of registering as a disabled person is one which the neurotic views with great suspicion. He sees himself labelled with a bad name and saddled with an additional handicap. If he is applying for a training course, the benefits of registration are obvious, as registered disabled persons are given priority of entry to the more popular courses, but if he is seeking a job he may feel under a cloud and just as liable to dismissal as if he were not registered. It is only after knowing the patient for some time and understanding why he reacts in his own particular way to the registration suggestion, that the D.R.O. can assess whether the question of registration is important in the patient's case or not. In practice it has been found that the best course to adopt has been to give the patient as much information as possible about the Disabled Persons (Employment) Act, and to discuss it with him both privately and at the patient discussion groups; at the latter he can hear a great variety of actual experiences from other patients, and in this way can be helped to make a decision for himself. If he prefers not to register, it is not necessarily a bad thing as it may mean that he does not need this support. If he does register he may quite easily be the sort of man who needs to use the Act as a target for his suppressed aggression.

'Working on the Unit, the D.R.O.s are given a definite role in a community which everyone recognizes as giving point and purpose to the psychiatric treatment, and a work goal to the man. This great advantage, together with the cumulative effect on the patient of the use of community and group methods of treatment—i.e. educational talks and the continual attempt by all the Unit staff to direct the patient's therapy towards a changed attitude to his future employment, should be borne in mind when considering the follow-up results of Unit patients and the control group.

'D.R.O.s at employment exchanges are working under entirely different conditions and do not have the constant opportunity of discussion with the psychiatrist and others interested in the resettlement of the unemployed neurotic. The only support and guidance the D.R.O. receives is on Form D.P.I.[1] and D.P.I.U.[2] It is not, therefore, surprising that the doctor, D.R.O. and unemployed neurotic often find it difficult to integrate constructively in an approach to an employment goal.'

The roles of the other important members of the Unit staff (the social workers and psychologist) are not treated separately here; as much attention is given to their roles as to the other staff groups, but there has been relatively less modification in their case than in the cases described. It is felt too, that the chapters written by them (Chapters VII, VIII and IX) deal in part with their separate roles.

---

[1] D.P.I is a form of report completed by hospital medical officers in respect of all hospital patients who will be discharged with residual disablement involving substantial handicap in getting or keeping employment. It is specially designed for use by D.R.O.s in their work of assisting the resettlement of disabled persons. It seeks to express residual capacity for work in terms which may be readily understood by laymen.

[2] D.P.I.U is a supplementary medical report for use in cases of psychiatric disorder. It is designed to give comprehensive medical guidance about the effects of psychiatric disorder in terms that the D.R.O. can interpret in relation to employment.

Up to now we have been discussing the staff roles, and in this section of the Unit community there has been a strong conscious urge to study and formulate such roles as an essential factor in the development of a therapeutic community. Clearly no such attitude motivates the behaviour of the patient community.

Patients

The role of the patient in the therapeutic community is more difficult to define than that of the various members of the staff. It is perhaps easier to think of it as an anticipated role. The aim is to help the patient to learn and accept his role in the Unit. The various social therapy techniques described in the next chapter may help this process as may the roles and role relationships of the doctors, nurses, and other members of the staff. As these roles are developed with a view to the maximum aid to the patient group one might describe the total culture as a therapeutic one. We attempt to give the patient some indication of his role even before he reaches hospital. Assuming that an application has been made for admission, and the patient has been put on the waiting list, a letter is sent to him telling him when he will be admitted; enclosed in the letter is an explanatory leaflet which reads as follows:

'This note is intended to explain to you what sort of place you are coming to. It is not a general hospital nor is it a mental hospital—it is a neurosis centre designed to help and treat patients whose psychological difficulties have led to some form of illness. There may be a physical aspect to your illness, and in such cases adequate facilities exist for proper medical treatment; most treatment here, however, centres around talks with your doctor. If you have problems to do with housing, pensions, ration books, etc., you can discuss these with the social worker. You may have had difficulty in finding work, or be dissatisfied with your present employment; in either case we would like to try and help you. As part of the treatment you will be expected to interest yourself in one of the workshops for two hours morning and afternoon; you will be shown these workshops on arrival, and will be free to choose whatever job interests you most. The workshops are for hairdressing, tailoring, plastering, bricklaying and carpentry for the male patients, and handicrafts and tailoring for the female patients. The workshops do not provide a training, but are intended to give you interesting work under conditions similar to those found in friendly, well-organized factories. We have found this type of occupation more useful in treating and rehabilitating our male patients than the more usual hospital occupation such as rug-making or leather work. Treatment also includes daily discussion groups, where an attempt is made to understand various psychological problems, and help you to a better understanding of your illness. You will find the nurses friendly and helpful and always available to talk to. Ample facilities exist for social activities such as indoor and outdoor games, dancing classes, socials, etc. If your doctor thinks you are well enough you will be granted a pass daily from hospital between the hours of 4 p.m. and 7 p.m., and on Wednesdays from 1 p.m. to 7 p.m.; week-end passes are from 9 a.m. Saturday to 7 p.m. Sunday. Patients must be in bed by 9 p.m. every night at which time the night nurses come on duty. We want to help you to get well, and, if you have employment difficulties, to help you get the right job. Patients are admitted for a trial period of two weeks, at the end of which time the situation is reviewed; the patient will then be informed by the doctor whether or not his case is considered to be suitable for further treatment in this hospital, or whether he would be better treated as an out-patient or referred back to his private doctor, and so on.'

The new patient is welcomed to the Unit by the nurses, and immediately introduced to a patient who has volunteered for this reception work as was described in Chapter II. The planned work day, and the ramification of the social life of the Unit, afford the new patient a wide range of roles from which he is largely free to choose for himself. Thus, he may choose the occupation which takes his fancy, and change this later if he wishes to do so; in the ward he may associate with whatever individual or group of individuals he wishes, or remain largely isolated. The majority of patients have had ample opportunity to play socially useful roles in the outside community had they been well enough to accept such roles, but they have frequently been forced into negative, passive or anti-social attitudes by their emotional difficulties. In the same way it is not enough to supply a pleasant and friendly environment for the patients while in hospital; an attempt must be made to understand their social difficulties and to master them. The skill of the nurses, and the value of the various social therapy techniques, can in part be assessed by their success in converting potential, into actual social and vocational roles which should, of course, be in conformity with the treatment aims of the Unit, and the needs of the individual patient. Moreover, if some of the patients have come to accept—at least in part—the Unit culture, then this factor may contribute to an individual patient's acculturation. In this sense it may be said that the role of the patient includes a potential therapeutic function in relation to other patients. Moreover, in some of the social therapy techniques patients are given the opportunity to contribute something to the treatment of other patients.

Our insistence that the whole day's programme must be considered as part of treatment, and that no patient is excused from attending the discussion groups, workshops, etc., forces the patient to participate in social situations; he may well resent this, but he is given the opportunity to ventilate his resentment in the group meetings. Group attitudes to familiar situations may be established at the group discussions, and tend to become established practice. Take the problem of the man who seeks advice from other patients regarding his own symptoms; he may arouse considerable anxiety in his fellow-patients by his talk, and they in turn may demand that discussion of such topics be forbidden. If at this stage an appeal were made to a staff member, the advice, if forthcoming, would in all probability be disregarded, and in any case any attempt on our part to limit or change the function or role of the patient or group of patients would be liable to misinterpretation. If the topic is arousing sufficient anxiety in the group, then it will probably be verbalized in the daily Unit discussion and the attitude of the group towards this topic may then change. Such attitudes tend to be perpetuated in the Unit community through its most stable, united and permanent group—i.e. the staff. The accumulation of such attitudes contributes to the Unit culture.

It might be said that the more the patient culture approximates to the Unit culture, as represented by the staff, the greater will be our effectiveness in treating new patients. In our opinion patients can usefully contribute to hospital treatment and all too often hospitals like prisons offer a harmful rather than a therapeutic culture to the new arrival.

In conclusion we would like to stress that the roles of the various personnel on the Unit are constantly changing and with it the culture of the group. In the early stages of our development the anxieties generated by the extremely difficult anti-social type of patient we had to handle, together with the need to protect our relatively young and inexperienced nursing staff who stay with us for only six to twelve months, led to a rather authoritarian type of régime. This is gradually changing and increasingly more responsibility is being taken from the doctor's role and transferred to the other personnel including the patients. Thus we are now testing out voluntary attendance at work therapy and the Unit discussion groups. However, development of this kind is hampered by our close proximity to the main hospital where a more orthodox authoritarian culture exists. The hospital administration, understandingly, resists too great differences between the two groups of patients.

CHAPTER IV

SOCIAL THERAPIES

GENERAL INTRODUCTION

IN a therapeutic community the whole of a patient's time spent in hospital is thought of as treatment. Treatment to be effective will not only involve the handling of the individual's neurotic problems, but also an awareness of the fresh problems which the fact of being in a neurosis hospital will create for the patient, and what aspects of the social situation can be used to aid treatment. The patient, the social *milieu* in which he lives and works, and the hospital community of which he becomes temporarily a member, are all important and interact on each other.

The term hospital has different meanings; its significance will vary according to its function (mental, general, etc.), and to the culture of the individual's group. The patient comes to hospital for many different reasons; in a general hospital he may, consciously at least, come to have his illness cured. His illness is something which he and his friends can conceptualize, and he enters hospital as naturally and as free from guilt as he would enter a restaurant. The neurosis centre, on the other hand, has as yet no such place in our cultural system; in the public mind it is probably more closely linked with a mental hospital than with a general hospital, and all the fears and prejudices associated with the former may be applied to it. Even more important, is the doubt which exists in the mind of the patient as to his right to fall ill; no one questions the right of a fracture patient to be ill and he is thus excused certain social obligations, but the neurotic can enjoy no such immunity.

What is meant by the terms health and illness is always difficult to define, but particularly so when we are thinking of the neurotic; by neurotic illness we mean emotional difficulties, conscious or unconscious, which result in an inability on the part of the individual to meet the needs of his environment, or to make adjustments (at a conscious or unconscious level) sufficient to maintain an adequate functional efficiency. What is meant by 'adequate' is open to many interpretations and is largely a subjective assessment; there is no doubt that the dividing line between health and illness is a very arbitrary one in the case of many neurotics. It can be said that the community resents the neurotic, and this applies even to the neurotic community itself, as Bion[1] has shown so clearly in his study of analytic groups. There are undoubtedly many factors involved in this hostility, and attitudes will vary with individuals; there seems, however, to be an almost universal tendency to think of the neurotic as escaping from his social obligations through illness, and this arouses various reactions including those of envy. The desire to escape from social commitments and seek a protected environment, such as we knew in infancy, is a daily experience in the life of everyone; any such turning away from reality on the part of the individual must be guarded against by a progressive community; and it is easier to withstand such temptations if we can project the guilt which they arouse on to someone else who has given up the struggle and become neurotically ill.

The patient himself may have many reasons, both conscious and unconscious, for coming to a neurosis centre. Consciously he may identify this type of hospital with a general hospital, and this is particularly true of ex-Forces personnel where Service psychiatry did much to educate public opinion, and neuroses became, in part at least, socially permissible. Much will depend on the nature of his illness and the reaction of his family and friends to it. However, there is good reason to think that the neurosis hospital appears in fantasy as a place where the neurotic's needs may be met. Any such hopes are soon dispelled on entering hospital as the neurotic realizes that many of the anxieties and social difficulties of his home environment are reproduced in this new community.

In war-time the situation was fundamentally different as one basic need at least could be satisfied; the need to escape from the anxieties represented by Army service was usually met by discharge from the Service. How little therapeutic value lay in this step alone, was shown by the results of Guttman's[2] follow-up study.

In most cases for the neurotic entering hospital there is some de-

---

[1] Bion, W. R., *Human Relations*, 3, 3, 1950.
[2] Guttman, E., *Report on Public Health and Medical Subjects*, No. 93, H.M. Stationery Office, 1946.

gree of guilt, and this mirrors the social censure which applies to the general public's attitude to this form of illness. He feels that he is giving in to his illness and is running away from his responsibilities; at the same time he may feel deeply wronged by society, and expects that in hospital he will at last be understood. All this emphasizes the complicated needs which the neurosis centre must attempt to meet. The first essential would appear to be that the trained staff working in such a centre should have a clear understanding of their various roles, and feel competent to meet them. We must face the fact, however, that no unanimity of opinion appears to exist on the question of the value of neurosis centres. Psychiatric opinion appears to be sharply divided on this issue the psychoanalysts tending to feel that it so complicates the transference situation, that much clinical research would need to be done and many new techniques evolved before they could have any positive attitude to the problem. Other psychiatrists rightly point out the danger of creating a sheltered environment, which may encourage regressive tendencies and make adjustment to reality even more difficult. Obviously, any discussion of in-patient neurosis centres must be guided by the organization of the particular centre. We believe that we are justified in treating our neurotics as in-patients, as the use of community techniques represents the most effective way of altering the anti-social attitudes of the type of patient we get, and for whom out-patient treatment methods would, we believe, be quite ineffective.

Unit Discussion Groups

The hundred patients belonging to the Industrial Neurosis Unit meet each week-day at 9 a.m. for a one-hour discussion on some sociological topic. The general programme has already been described in Chapter II. On two mornings a week a discussion group is held, usually taken by one of the doctors, but not infrequently by another staff member (psychiatric social worker, nurse, disablement resettlement officer, psychologist), or even a guest speaker. The nurses on duty are usually present. The discussion is opened by a short talk on some sociological problem followed by a discussion in which there is usually a large degree of participation. The problem raised is always one which bears directly on the life of the ordinary working man; thus domestic problems such as: 'Should marriage partners work?'—'Should husband and wife spend their leisure together?', or various problems relating to the upbringing of children, attitude to authority, etc., are discussed. The content of the talks with which the speaker opens the discussion is left largely to the individual concerned; he may talk once a week for three months and then be relieved by someone else. The role of the doctor in these Unit discussion groups has already been discussed in the previous chapter. Different doctors employ different methods and the technique employed by any one doctor may vary considerably from time to time. Thus discussion alone, various forms of spontaneous acting, a reproduction of a psychiatric out-patient department[1] with the doctor playing his own role and a nurse portraying the role of an actual out-patient, and a problem family,[2] have all been used. The most important thing is to arouse the patient's interest and if possible his active participation so that he changes from a passive or defeatist attitude and actually tests out the possibility of change in his real life problems.

Familiar emotional problems are touched on and the individual responds according to his own particular pattern; in the discussion he realizes that there are other possible ways of reacting, some of which may allow him greater opportunity for abreaction or for instinctual gratification. At the same time there is frequently a form of group attitude apparent which may influence the individual in his choice of behaviour. Our impression is that the 'work' of the meeting is done largely at a feeling level and there is very little gain in insight for the majority of patients. Certainly the meetings are a social experience; the small crowded room, the daily meetings, the absence of unfamiliar faces and the general permissive atmosphere, are an invitation to free speech and emotional responses. In many of the patients, response will be largely, if not entirely inhibitory, while in others will be aroused all the individual's rebelliousness against the group or, it may be, against the doctor. These situations must be faced and, if possible, worked through, although inevitably many people will remain dissatisfied by the end of the meeting; they will go on discussing the problem with their friends or the nurses and may later revive the topic in a small therapeutic group or in individual psychotherapeutic interviews with the doctor.

Despite the incompleteness of these meetings, an opportunity is afforded for the expression of emotionally toned ideas within a group under relatively controlled circumstances. The whole atmosphere

[1] Jones, M., *Brit. Med. Jour.*, 1, 756, 1949.
[2] Jones, M., *Amer. Jour. Psychiat.*, 101, 292, 1944.

tends to be more emotionally charged than in the small therapeutic groups, where there is much greater cohesiveness and a better opportunity to work through a situation with gain in insight. The discussion group is more permissive in the sense that, as one of a large crowd of patients, the individual is in less direct contact with the doctor, and is more ready to reproduce his own particular emotional patterns. We feel that there is some gain in reproducing these reactions which can be discussed with perhaps some increase of objective awareness on the part of the patient; but the main value is probably from comparison of an individual's reaction with those of other members of the group, and above all, an awareness of what pattern appears to meet with the greatest approval from the group. We believe that all this can have a socializing value, as whatever the dynamics may be, the most rebellious or inhibited patient is subjected to a group experience, and the group does literally include all these divergent types in its loosely knit but nevertheless real structure. The doctor must of course avoid, if possible, becoming emotionally involved, or at least he must not show that he is; daily experience of this type of benign authority has probably got considerable value, especially in view of the fact that most of our patients come from broken homes where parents all too frequently have expressed their anxiety in intolerance and aggression directed towards their children.

The various doctors taking these discussion groups use different approaches according to their beliefs and personalities, but the general pattern of the meeting is the same. Dr. Merry is relatively active in his handling of the community, and the following report is written by him and describes one such meeting.

'One morning the subject suggested was marriage. A Mr. F. opened the discussion. He was a single man aged twenty-five, and had come to this country as a refugee from Germany at the age of fourteen. He was a tactless man with a jarring voice, and had little inhibition. He would interrupt and attempt to join in small discussion groups without invitation, and he would air his views very volubly at the slightest provocation. At this period he was very unpopular with the group, and the group expressed their feelings about him in no uncertain fashion. Mr. F. droned on and on in his high-pitched, irritating voice. Patients became restless, began to whisper and cough, and mimicked his foreign accent. After about ten minutes one of the mimics, a Mr. T., stood up and protested very forcibly against the stupidity of Mr. F. who was a single man and therefore knew nothing about marriage. Mr. T., an aggressive psychopath, aged forty-nine, had been married to an epileptic who was certified and had been in a mental hospital for sixteen years. For the last fourteen years he had been living with another woman who had adopted his name, and there was a twelve-year-old son resulting from this union. "Mrs." T. had informed me that Mr. T. was an egocentric, irritable and aggressive man, who was very cruel to his son. She had urged Mr. T. to get a divorce from his wife and marry her, but he had seen no reason to take this step. His egocentricity and his aggression had driven her to direct more and more attention and affection to her son. She was very dissatisfied with the present domestic state, and was determined that when he left hospital their relationship would cease. At individual interviews Mr. T. confirmed most of his wife's utterances in one way or another, but would never admit to a sadistic attitude towards his son. Mr. T. continued to taunt and mimic Mr. F. unmercifully. I intervened and suggested that Mr. T. was attacking Mr. F. for reasons other than that he was ignorant of marriage. Mr. T. denied this and was most indignant at the suggestion that he was being at all hostile. I informed the group that I knew of Mr. F.'s unpopularity and suggested that we discuss this unpleasant situation. Showers of reasons for his unpopularity were poured forth. He was arrogant, he was voluble, he was tactless and so on. I suggested that although these reasons were perhaps valid, there might be other mechanisms at work. I then went on to discuss aggression and hate.

'Aggression and hate were emotions, which if indeed not inborn, were present at a very early stage of our development. We loved and hated the same people at different times, e.g. our parents. We repressed our hate for our parents because it was "bad" to hate and also because our hate might result in reprisals. However, there was a strong need to express this aggressive urge. We could all be much more pleasant to our loved ones if we could work off our hate on somebody or something else, e.g. a subordinate or a political or national enemy. At all times we were searching for a whipping boy in order to vent our aggression "legitimately". Were not Mr. F. in the hospital, then sooner or later the group would have found another object for their hostility. The presence of a focus for hate facilitated the expression of goodwill and comradeship amongst the haters.

'I continued and pointed out that Mr. F. was a foreigner who spoke with an accent. He was different from the rest of the group. He was strange—a danger. The group always united against strangers to combat them more effectively. Were not Mr. F. a German then his shortcomings would not have been so disturbing to the group. He might have been unpopular, but not so unpopular as he was in fact now. I informed the group of what little I knew of Mr. F.'s background. He had felt rejected by his parents and had obviously been rejected by his father-country. He had always felt unwanted and was apparently not very welcome in our group. True, he was not a personality who was easily acceptable—he seemed to be deliberately provoking hostility as if he had a need to recreate this pattern of rejection. Perhaps his arrogance, his volubility, his tactlessness, were a result of frantic efforts to obtain acceptance by society, but his unconscious need to be rejected was stronger than his conscious desire to be accepted. I concluded my contribution with the injunction that we should always question our motives in any action which might cause even the slightest unhappiness to others. There was unhappiness enough in the world without thoughtless and unnecessary contributions. It is understood that we all lost our tempers and were cruel at one time or another, but on these occasions we must recognize and accept the fact that in most cases we are looking for an opportunity to vent our aggression. When I had finished there was complete silence. There was no verbal contribution from the group and I walked out through the silent room. As I left the room, the unusually long silence was broken by prolonged and vigorous clapping of greater intensity than usually accompanied the end of a session.

'I made my way to my clinic and had not been there five minutes when there was a knock on the door and in walked Mr. T. He was obviously disturbed and near to tears. He hoped that I had not really thought that he had been deliberately cruel to Mr. F. and he had not meant to be malicious with his taunts. He had not realized that he was making anybody unhappy. Spontaneously he suggested that perhaps he had been unwittingly cruel to his own son in this fashion. I reassured him that I was certain that he was not being deliberately cruel to either Mr. F. or his son, and I suggested that in future his attempts at humour might have less venom now that he realized the possible effects his behaviour might have on others.

'Some days later I was stopped by Mr. F. who thanked me for discussing his problem openly. He had noticed a marked change in the attitude of the group towards him. They were more friendly and tolerant and seemed to be accepting him more readily. On questioning a number of patients including Mr. T., a week after this session, they confirmed Mr. F.'s observation that he was being absorbed into the group, but they maintained that this was because Mr. F. had changed. He was not as rude, tactless, or voluble as formerly. It was not *they* who had changed. They had never really disliked him in the first instance.

'For the rest of his stay in hospital Mr. F. became more and more incorporated in the group, though it could not be said that he was ever very popular. It would be a fair comment to say that the group had accepted his shortcomings and made some allowance for them. It is interesting to know that nine months after his discharge from hospital Mr. T. was very well. He was working as a navvy although there was no financial necessity for him to work at all. His "wife" informed me that she was most satisfied with the behaviour of her "husband" in general and towards her son in particular.'

A very different technique is adopted by Dr. Baker. For example, in attempting to assess the patient's attitude to work, to our compulsory work therapy, and to the workshops themselves, he handled the meeting as follows. When the whole patient population and staff had assembled he asked one of the Workshop Instructors, Mr. S., to play the role of a new patient. He then enacted an interview with Mr. S. and asked him what occupation he would like while in hospital. Mr. S. said he had seen all the workshops but that nothing there interested him. After a pause Dr. Baker turned to the patients and asked what he was to do now. Several suggestions were immediately forthcoming which Dr. Baker then put to Mr. S., but without any success; all Mr. S. was interested in was doing some clerical work—if we hadn't that then he did not want any occupation at all. Again Dr. Baker turned to the patients for guidance. They now wished to know if Mr. S. had ever *tried* to use his hands, had he difficulty in concentration or did he easily become bored. Mr. S. did not change his attitude. 'Shall we let him off occupations altogether?' asked Dr. Baker. A chorus of 'No!' greeted this inquiry. The patients then went on to elaborate how, if left to himself, Mr. S. would just drift. Mr. S. remarked, 'I came here for treatment. I need a rest not work.' (Cheers from the audience.) However, the patients insisted that he would be better fully occupied and asked if he realized that it was not an eight-hour day they worked but only four hours. Mr. S. now asked 'Why should I work?' The patients remarked on the need for everyone to work, not only for financial reasons but for their own mental health. Dr. Baker then explained the staff attitude towards work therapy and went on to ask the patients how real conditions of work in hospital should be made—should they be like a factory so that everyone must arrive on time or be discharged? The patients pointed out that if they felt they had *got* to go to work then it tended to antagonize them. Dr. Baker then asked how he could round off his interview with Mr. S. The patients advised that Mr. S. should have a week's trial in one of the workshops after which he could then discuss the problem again with his doctor.

Dr. Baker now asked the new patients in the group to stand up and introduce themselves. All six had arrived the day before and had been shown around the workshops and had met their doctors for an initial interview. One of these new patients was asked to take the place of Mr. S. Mr. W., a patient with a long record of unemployment, did so. Dr. Baker now turned to the patients and asked what sort of questions he should put to Mr. W. Having been briefed he asked Mr. W. what his last job had been. Mr. W. said he had done heavy work in the engineering trade but had had to give it up. 'Why did you find it difficult?' asked the doctor. Mr. W. replied that it had been dull and boring so he had tried other work but it had always been the same story. Dr. Baker asked again, 'Well, what would you like to do here?' Mr. W. replied, 'I don't want to do anything.' Dr. Baker then turned to the patients one of whom suggested that Mr. W. should be allowed to wander around the workshops where he would probably settle down in one. Another, however, pointed out that Mr. W. had been around once, and if after further wandering he still did not settle, we had the same problem. Another suggested that the community should find out what his interests were because maybe he wanted a job where he could use his brain as well as his hands. So Dr. Baker put these questions to Mr. W. who replied 'Yes, I've been a fur dresser and I liked that.' 'And why did you give that up?' asked Dr. Baker. Mr. W. replied, 'Because I liked night work and when that ended I did not like the same job on the day shift. I don't like mixing with people.' A patient then suggested that we should place him in one of the workshops in the morning and send him to the local Government training centre at Waddon in the afternoon where he could be tried out in a trade. Dr. Baker remarked, 'But we don't yet know if he is suited for a trade.' A patient now stated, 'We don't usually send new patients to Waddon —he might not be suited for it temperamentally.' Another patient suggested that physical training was the best activity we had. Dr. Baker asked Mr. W. about physical training but the latter replied that he would not last an hour at this. Dr. Baker then asked another patient, Mr. C., who had been in hospital for some time, to come out and explain the work therapy to Mr. W. The latter was told that he ought to mix more with other people at work. Mr. W. replied, 'But I don't want to mix with other people.' Mr. C. answered this with, 'You meet people at the local, don't you?' 'Don't go to pubs,' said Mr. W. bluntly. Mr. C. responded with, 'Well, I suggest that you just go and look at the occupation shops for a week.' 'I always keep myself to myself,' Mr. W. stubbornly replied. Mr. C. said in explanation, 'That's part of your neurosis. You must give things a trial and try to change, for after all you can keep yourself to yourself even in the workshops.' Dr. Baker thanked Mr. C. who returned to his seat in the audience. A patient now queried, 'Does he want to mix with people?' Mr. W. replied, 'I'll mix but I won't talk, but if an argument starts then I'll join in.' A patient questioned, 'Is he afraid of talking in case he makes a fool of himself?' Dr. Baker suggested, 'Well, go ahead and ask him.' Mr. W. agreed that there might be something in this. 'Perhaps he's learnt he gets people's backs up when he talks,' suggested another patient. Dr. Baker agreed that the discussion related Mr. W.'s work difficulties to his personality defects and that if these could be remedied it would be much easier for Mr. W. to find satisfactory employment. He went on to point out that Mr. W. had already taken an active part in the community life of the Unit by his performance, that he had been given an opportunity to talk without being misunderstood or being laughed at, that perhaps he would go on improving.

In conclusion Dr. Baker pointed out that there was general agreement that no one liked the idea of being compelled to work. Indeed, many patients were over-sensitive to any suggestion of compulsion. This was related to experiences in their early lives when compelled to do things to please an aggressive father or over-anxious mother. The patients were encouraged to review their past work history and their patterns of behaviour which had led to failure, and then to use our workshop facilities to try and create new and healthier patterns.

Psychodrama

This technique has been employed since January 1944 when we were at Mill Hill Emergency Hospital. The procedure consists of dramatized episodes from a patient's past life. A patient volunteers to present his problem as he sees it in this play form; he chooses his own cast from the patient community or from the nurses, and may or may not seek help in the writing and production of the play. It takes a week to produce and the personnel are excused from occupations for this period. As might be expected there are tremendous variations in the quality and range of the productions, but frequently a surprisingly high standard is achieved. The play usually takes about half an hour to perform, and is attended by the entire patient population, staff and visitors. Following the production a discussion takes place under the directorship of one of the doctors (usually the doctor of the patient who has put on his psychodrama). The patients participate freely in the discussion and the doctor seldom says anything until the end of the meeting when he attempts to sum up what has been said, and amplifies it to bring out any particular point he may wish to express. During the discussion, some of Moreno's[1] techniques of spontaneous acting may be used to see how the patient would behave in certain theoretical situations, and so on. The whole meeting lasts about one hour.

The value of psychodrama can be discussed from three points of view; the patient himself, the production group (which of course, includes the patient), and the audience.

In reliving incidents from his past life the patient has to give considerable thought to the characters whom he is portraying in addition to his own central role. In the process of writing and production he frequently sees aspects of the total situation which escaped him on the original occasion; in a sense he has to identify himself with each character in turn in order to be able to write a psychodrama at all. Clearly, ample opportunity is afforded to him to distort the various characters according to his own prejudices and neurotic difficulties, and the psychodrama can be used by the patient largely to satisfy his own inner needs; thus the patient may use his psychodrama to demonstrate his unworthiness to the group or it may be that he uses

---

[1] Moreno, J. L. (1946), *Psychodrama*. Beacon House, N.Y.

the situation to show how deeply he has been wronged by society. The week spent on rehearsals and the actual production itself may afford an excellent opportunity for emotional abreaction. Patients have frequently remarked that they felt considerable relief of tension following the production of their story. The psychodrama also affords an opportunity to achieve mastery in a situation or situations which in real life had overwhelmed the patient. For instance, a young man of nineteen years who had marked social anxiety which prevented him from mixing even in the sheltered environment of the Unit, was asked if he would care to produce his psychodrama; at first the idea terrified him and he literally shrank from the thought of ever having to speak in public, partly because he had a severe stammer since early childhood. For the first few weeks he was given the job of curtain pulling or scene shifting, and then he himself offered to speak some lines if he could not be seen by the audience; on this first trial he stammered occasionally at rehearsals, but at the actual performance he was surprised when he spoke without difficulty. After a few more weeks he was again invited to produce his own life story and it only needed a little encouragement from some of his fellow-patients to make him agree. In the early stages of writing, deciding on details of production, etc., he was tense and unsettled. He sought the Secretary's help in the production and she found him so restless at this stage that the preliminary work was done walking in the hospital grounds. He improved progressively as the production got under way and finally lost his stammer completely; in fact some new members who were introduced at a late stage in the rehearsals wondered whose problem they were enacting. The patient was enormously pleased by his performance and had a feeling of real accomplishment.

So far we have made no serious attempt to extend the psycho-dramatic technique to achieve uncovering therapy; we believe that from the patient's point of view the technique is essentially supportive. The patient's defences are strengthened and some of his attitudes may change, but there is no real insight into his emotional problems. It is surprising the degree of support which a patient usually obtains not only from the cast, but also from the whole audience. His problem becomes known to everyone on the Unit, and inevitably his position in the community is altered, usually in the direction of a more sympathetic understanding from the other people.

The psychodrama affords an opportunity for the formation of a small group with a positive goal. The patient who volunteers to put on a psychodrama chooses his own cast (usually six to eight people) and these people usually resemble the real characters he wishes to portray. The tendency is, of course, for him to choose his cast from amongst his friends. Not infrequently tension develops in this drama group largely focused around the central character, but on the whole the cast shows an extraordinary tolerance towards the main participant. For instance, in one psychodrama a young man with a severe character disorder chose a dominating fellow-patient to play the role of his father. The real father had been an alcoholic who later became schizophrenic; he had treated the patient very cruelly as a child, and in real life the patient had never lifted a hand to his father who simply terrified him. During rehearsals, on two consecutive occasions, re-enactment of a scene where his father had forcibly pushed him, led to an uncontrolled attack on the patient playing the role of his father. The patient concerned took this in good part although physically injured, but after discussion with the group it was agreed that the psychodrama should be altered to avoid this provocation.

Despite the tensions aroused the psychodramatic group never seems to give up, and a production appears every Friday. To the other members of the cast the psychodrama offers an excellent opportunity to play a useful social role. The rehearsals proceed daily for a week, the time spent being two hours in the morning and two hours in the afternoon.

The audience is only concerned with the actual psychodramatic production, but they participate freely in the active discussion which invariably follows the psychodrama. Frequently members of the audience are asked to come out on the stage and act out some situation which they have been discussing, along with the appropriate members of the cast; this procedure seems to add much more than does a mere verbal contribution. Individuals in the audience inevitably identify themselves with the characters in the play, and adopt certain attitudes. In the discussion which follows the psychodrama these attitudes are contrasted with those of other participants. Moreover, at times a group attitude appears to emerge. The individual is afforded an opportunity to compare his attitude with that of other people and of the group, and we believe that in this setting certain attitudes may be altered. The whole group also feels itself to be participating in a treatment situation, the end in view being to help a fellow-patient.

The group has definitely changed during the years we have been using a dramatic technique; the attitude now is one of much greater responsibility than formerly towards the person whose problem is being dramatized, and the group participation in the discussion afterwards is correspondingly greater. This suggests the development of a group technique which is accepted as a legitimate medium for the expression of personal problems. The plays usually raise very intimate questions and often invite censure; the fact that great tolerance and understanding are invariably shown must help to restore social confidence, not only in the individual directly concerned, but in all the patients who have identified themselves with their fellow-patient.

In addition to the social therapies described above there is a wider cultural aspect of treatment. Adam Curle[1] in his most interesting follow-up study of ex-civilian resettlement unit personnel says that 'culture may be considered as a cluster of socially determined attitudes and behaviour patterns grouped and elaborated round structurally defined roles and relationships.

'Culture may be said to work by providing the individual with a series of techniques through which he may regulate and enrich his social relationships.'

Curle believes that it is the internal assimilation and integration of culture that is primarily disturbed in the process of desocialization of ex-P.o.W. personnel. This would appear to be largely true in the case of our chronic unemployed population. It would also be true to say that we have made great efforts to develop a suitable hospital culture in an attempt to resocialize the patients. The weekly consideration and discussion of the therapeutic role of each staff member within the community, the attempt to become aware of group tensions and deal with them, the attention to free communication between the various patient and staff groups, and the educational discussion groups all aim at helping the patient to find a satisfactory role in the hospital community.

Another factor in aiding this process of assimilation within the Unit culture is the emphasis on jobs, the prestige given to this goal by the staff (particularly the nurses), and the attempt made to give

[1] Adam Curle, *Human Relations*, 1, 42, 1947.

the patient a vocational role while still in hospital. As already stated there is no 'occupational therapy' as is commonly understood in hospital practice and we prefer the term 'work therapy'; the Unit workshops aim at a normal factory environment so that the man is being prepared for the type of unskilled vocational role which he might follow in normal life. If he has any particular abilities as shown by vocational testing, or more important, shows a real desire to work, he may be sent on trial to the local Government training centre where he can try out a trade, being treated as just another trainee although still in hospital. Alternatively he can be tried out in a local firm, and to date over thirty employers have helped us in this way. This emphasis on the vocational role in people who have been unemployed for some time has probably a strong socializing influence. But the resistances to work are very strong in some patients and there are times when the 'healthy' attitude towards work is largely absent in the group. It is in just this sort of situation that the attitude of the staff is so important in maintaining the group culture. In general, such situations are met by a free discussion of the problems with the patients and separately with the staff. It is usually possible to get some insight into the dynamics of the situation although frequent meetings may be necessary. But although such fluctuations are constantly occurring it is surprising how consistently the general cultural outlook is maintained despite an intake of about ten new admissions per week.

There is a tendency towards the development of a more involved culture—take for instance the psychodramas, which have been held every week since the inception of the Unit: at first the writer remained anonymous or claimed that the characters were fictitious; more recently the patient has appeared in his own role and frequently displays many intimate facts relating to his past life. Such a development suggests a changing group culture and a growing willingness on the part of the individual patient to trust the community and look to it for help. It is surprising how quickly new patients seem to accept this pattern of behaviour, and talk and act with a freedom unknown in their previous lives.

Other social activities such as beginners' dancing classes, socials, concerts, etc., are not discussed here because they are familiar activities in any well-run psychiatric unit. The important point is that they should be attended by the Unit staff and conceived of as part of treatment, affording excellent opportunities for creating social roles, and a natural relationship between patients and staff.

After discharge from hospital a patient who lives in the London area may attend the social club which we run in the centre of London by courtesy of St. George's Hospital. This club meets one evening a week and is always attended by several members of the staff, so that contact may be maintained with the Unit even after discharge from hospital. In addition all the doctors have out-patient sessions in various teaching hospitals in London so that ex-patients can be given continued support if this is considered necessary.

CHAPTER V

SOME PROBLEMS OF IN-PATIENT PSYCHOTHERAPY IN A NEUROSIS UNIT

BY DR. THOMAS FREEMAN

A HOSPITAL dealing exclusively with psychoneurotics, has resulted from the necessity of coping with the ever increasing
number of emotionally sick individuals. Until recently, the
psychoneurotic patient found himself in a difficult situation when he
came to look for treatment. If he was well-to-do he had the option
of either out-patient therapy, or he could enter one of the many
private psychiatric hospitals which cater for the neurotic and psychotic patient. If he was unfortunate enough to lack sufficient means, he
had to content himself with visits to his general practitioner. If his
condition was more severe, then he could apply to one of the mental
hospitals for admission as a voluntary patient. In many instances he
may have been able to attend an out-patient psychiatric department
at one of the more progressive general hospitals. To-day this state of
affairs has greatly altered for the better, and there are several neurosis
centres in the United Kingdom. On the Industrial Neurosis Unit at
Belmont Hospital, we are attempting to apply psychotherapeutic
methods of treatment, but are meeting with tremendous difficulties.
Firstly, the type of patient we admit—mostly severe character disorders with poorly integrated personalities—does not offer good
material for psychoanalysis or for any form of psychotherapy. Then
the patients stay in hospital for an average of four months, and each
doctor has a case load of twenty to thirty patients, so that no time is
available to apply a psychoanalytic technique to more than one or
two selected patients. Finally, the problem of psychotherapy for in-
patients is fundamentally different to the treatment of out-patients.
These treatment difficulties are discussed in this paper and particular
attention paid to the complications which arise when treatment is
carried out on hospital patients.

There is quite an extensive literature on the subject of in-patient
psychiatric treatment with special reference to psychotherapy. All

69

this work has come from private institutions where the patient population consists of psychotics and those severe neuroses and character disorders, which preclude out-patient treatment. In the private hospital, patients can be kept as long as necessary even when the clinical condition is no longer acute. The medical and nursing staff can be regulated in accordance with the number of patients, and the type of treatment employed in the hospital. W. C. Menninger (1936) describes this favourable environment where fifty patients are under the care of ten full-time physicians. Such conditions do not exist in a psychoneurosis hospital where the State assumes responsibility for the patient's welfare. The need for economy, the large number of patients, and the relative scarcity of psychiatrists do not permit a free application of the recommendations made by various writers in this field.

Under such conditions it is easy to understand the tendency of many psychiatrists to turn to physical methods of treatment in the hope of quick and successful results. The war years popularized such therapies as modified insulin, continuous narcosis, and the chemical abreactive techniques. Initially introduced to treat the acute and subacute war neuroses they were soon applied to all forms of neurotic illness. They have not maintained their early promise, and this is perhaps more comprehensible in the light of the different clinical material to be dealt with at the present time.

Is the psychological approach in a better position to offer help to the psychiatrist? Knight (1945), one of the first psychiatrists to use analytic psychotherapy within a hospital believes that it can. He recognizes the difficulty of thoroughly applying a treatment programme based on psychoanalytic principles in hospitals, where the patient–psychiatrist, patient–nurse ratio is high but nevertheless does not think it out of the question for these principles to be applied in a modified degree in the larger hospitals, where conditions are not so favourable. What are these principles to which Knight refers? They are based on a psychoanalytic understanding of patients' behaviour while under hospitalization.

W. C. Menninger (1936) formulates therapeutic aims in line with the two major instinctual drives postulated by Freud, the sexual and aggressive. Menninger believes that the symptoms and the behaviour of neurotic and psychotic patients, represent disturbances in the proper fusion and expression of these instincts. He describes 'devices' to correct disturbances in the sexual and aggressive drives.

He considers it necessary for the medical director, the psychiatrist and the nurses, not only to have the accepted psychiatric background, but they must have special training in psychoanalysis, and so be able to administer to the unconscious needs of the patients as expressed in their symptoms and behaviour.

Papers of this type are based directly on the theory and practice of psychoanalysis. This is the source of another difficulty. The majority of psychiatrists have no first-hand experience of psychoanalysis, and as a result the recommendations made by many workers have only a theoretical interest. The psychiatrist would like to be helped in his daily hospital work by psychoanalysis, but the absence of psychoanalytically trained psychiatrists makes this almost impossible. The presence of such workers imparts an interest and an atmosphere, which allows the non-analytically trained psychiatrists to participate more fully in the psychotherapeutic activity.

Karl Menninger (1940) says, 'We have not found it essential that a psychiatrist be analysed in order to acquire such an attitude . . .', i.e. an attitude which looks for an unconscious motivation in the behaviour of the patient. He believes that the 'proper attitude can be taught and furthermore it is contagious, it can be caught. Young psychiatrists quickly absorb the spirit and philosophy that permeates an institution. . . '. Rickman (1948) similarly discusses the application of psychoanalysis in the psychiatric hospital. He emphasizes the importance of the transference situation, and the possibility of the patient's behaviour being understood through its manifestations. He does not consider any aspect of in-patient treatment to be incompatible with analytic therapy, provided that every event is referred back to the transference situation. These papers imply the employment of psychoanalysts in addition to the regular medical staff. However desirable this may be, the present situation invalidates the very real advances advocated in these articles.

In the psychoneurosis hospital the patients are not physically ill; they can get about and are not restricted in any way. Facilities for social activities are given high priority, and various other recreations are provided apart from occupational or work therapy. Men and women patients can mix freely. Most patients are rather timid and shy at first, but they soon settle down. For better or worse, they are forced to accept one another's company. This is very difficult for some patients and they reactively develop anxiety and other anomalous responses.

Most patients come to hospital with the conscious hope of a complete cure, naïvely convinced that the power of cure lies in the doctors' hands; unfortunately this hope is not always fulfilled. Each patient can only remain in hospital a limited time, this is usually about three to six months, although there is no restriction on a patient remaining longer than this. Whatever the attitude of the administration on this question, and however liberal it may be, the psychiatrist is forced to limit the patient's stay if he is not to find himself with thirty or more patients to treat. Such a situation results in a complete breakdown of therapeutic endeavours.

The fact of the patients being resident in hospital, introduces a new complication not to be found with out-patient treatment. This is to be seen in the attitude the patient adopts to hospitalization. One group of patients tends to be very co-operative, obedient and if anything over-submissive. They are always on their best behaviour. They feel very keenly their dependence on the hospital, and as a rule they hold the medical staff in the highest esteem. It is no easy matter to get them to act naturally as they would at home. This group abhor the idea of being angry, discontented or irritable with the doctors or nurses, and they readily express their disapproval of those who voice such sentiments. Only after some time do these patients express themselves naturally, and under an authoritarian régime, their real behaviour would never be observed. The other group are quite different. They are unconcerned about the hospital regulations, they have apparently no regard for the efforts made on their behalf, and they continually criticize everything which is not to their liking. These patients stand out in relief in comparison with those of the former group. All gradations of behaviour exist, ranging from the pure culture of each type, to intermediate varieties.

Psychoanalysts have principally contributed to the understanding of this behaviour in hospital. They have demonstrated the tendency of patients, when placed in a new environment, to relive past emotional experiences in terms of the present. Simmel (1929) explains that the patient's attitude in the hospital, is merely a reflection of his behaviour outside. The family situation is re-enacted within the hospital structure, the patient playing the part he did in childhood. Simmel emphasizes the extension of the doctor-patient relationship beyond the consulting room, in attempting to comprehend many aspects of patients' behaviour. He points out that the in-patient is far more inclined to act out his mental conflicts, than the out-patient. The hospital patient is always trying to avoid directing his hostility to the doctor, and instead usually displaces it on to other members of the medical and nursing staff. This attempt by the patient to play off one member of the staff against another, is to be constantly guarded against. Other writers, for example Bullard (1940), similarly describe the reactions of patients who are being treated by psychoanalysis in hospital. If buried emotional reactions are to be disclosed by analytic therapy, then it is inevitable that there will be repercussions outside the consulting room.

In hospitals described by the psychoanalytic writers, the doctor sees the patient for an hour a day. This arrangement is only changed when the patient is psychotic, and then not invariably. In such instances the analytic technique is considerably modified. Fromm-Reichmann (1947) attaches considerable importance to the psychotherapist joining in as a part of the therapeutic community. She feels he ought to participate in the hospital activities even at the expense of his time with individual patients. He ought to make ward rounds, visit the occupational shops, and join in social functions. This alteration in the role of the psychoanalyst is no doubt dictated by the type of patient treated in her hospital.

In the psychoneurosis hospital time is the vital factor. Even if there were psychoanalytically trained psychiatrists on the staff, a case load of twenty or more patients make it impossible to spend five or even four hours a week with one individual. There are a few patients whose illness would respond excellently to analytic therapy, for example anxiety and conversion hysterias, mild obsessional neuroses, etc. The only way of dealing with this mass of clinical material seems to be by a selection of cases; this is what invariably happens in practice.

The psychotherapy employed acknowledges the limitation imposed upon it by the patient's short stay in hospital. After a formal history-taking, the patient is allowed to unfold his story as he likes. He is not limited to talking of the history of his illness, but is encouraged to discuss any aspect of his life. This method is not very successful with those patients who find difficulty in talking. These are the cases who require much more time than is available for them, but in actual fact no unit psychiatrist can devote more than three or four half-hours a week to any patient. Even so the psychiatrist gets to know quite a lot about the patient if the treatment is continued over five or six months. An alternative approach is to attack the symptoms directly as in the classical cathartic therapy introduced by Breuer and Freud (1895). In this treatment memories and often some of the determinants of the illness are revealed.

The present-day exponents of catharsis induce the patient, with the aid of various chemical agents, to abreact. They lay emphasis on the general emotional release, apart from the recovery of traumatic episodes. These therapists ignore the fact that a particular emotional attitude may serve as a defence against a deeper fear which is unconscious. Equally significant is the fact that catharsis is in practice divorced from the patient's relationships within the hospital. The material obtained during catharsis is not linked up with the patient's life in hospital or his life outside.

The following case illustrates some of these points. A woman patient of thirty-two years, was admitted to hospital with a history of having suffered from vomiting for the past six years. She was allowed to talk freely and spent the first twenty sessions expressing the most intense hostility against her father. She insisted that she had hardly ever thought of her father until she commenced treatment. As the patient continued, it became apparent that the hostility had at least two purposes. It prevented the emergence of her love for her father which he had rejected most cruelly in her childhood. This belief that the hate concealed love, was supported by her kind and thoughtful behaviour in hospital toward an older, almost destitute male patient, who was clearly a father substitute for her. Secondly, the aggression covered anxiety. This anxiety came from her childhood fear of her father, the fear that her father would discover her chance knowledge of his sexual activities. The symptom of vomiting was intimately related to her feelings of disgust when she encountered traces of her father's sexual activities. Her younger siblings were able to exploit her guilt about the secret even although they did not know about it themselves. In the cathartic therapy, the hate would have been abreacted without any attempt to understand the mechanism of the patient's behaviour.

Simmel's observation that patients attempt to avoid the transference reaction is particularly important. This avoidance is particularly obvious with the first group of patients described above. The fact that the patient is only seen three times a week allows him sufficient opportunity to hide his transference reactions behind the account of daily activities, which are always faithfully reported. This may not be a very difficult problem for the experienced psychoanalyst, but for many psychiatrists the doctor-patient relationship soon becomes hazy and vague.

This type of situation occurred with a young woman patient of twenty-four years who was admitted to the hospital because of depression and anxiety dreams. By allowing the girl to talk freely it soon became evident that her symptoms had been precipitated by the upsurge of sexual feeling accompanying the onset of an attachment to a young man. She was very disturbed by the sexual impulses which she did not welcome in herself. Under the influence of the positive transference, her symptoms soon cleared up. From then on the treatment made no further progress. She avoided the transference relationship successfully, and it was never really possible to know what her emotional attitude to the psychiatrist was, or what behaviour she was repeating from the past. She maintained a façade of alternating cheerfulness and depression. This behaviour in treatment, contrasted with her activity in the hospital where she always appeared bright, energetic and sociable. The only trace of what was possibly a displacement of the transference feelings, was her flirtation with two patients. This patient was able to isolate her relationship to the doctor from the rest of her behaviour in the hospital. She was able to sidetrack the task of understanding something of her problem through the medium of the transference situation. Perhaps patients unconsciously or consciously divine that they will not be permitted to complete an understanding of their illness, and subsequently refuse to become involved in such an unsatisfactory situation.

Short-term psychotherapy is unable radically to alter the patient's personality in the light of the early childhood neurosis. However, these early problems are reflected in the patient's everyday behaviour in the present. The material obtained from the patient in the space of three or four months, is sometimes sufficient to throw light on one or more behaviour patterns, which the patient uses in life situations. Occasionally these patterns become clear in the transference situation. In other instances observation of the patient's relationships in the hospital, supplies equally important information.

An example of this was provided by another woman patient of twenty-six years, who complained of severe headaches. She was married but unfortunately was completely frigid, so that her relations with her husband left much to be desired. Although genital sexuality was repugnant to her, she was nevertheless very fond of male company. From the moment she arrived in hospital she enjoyed herself, attending the patients' dances and socials, and making herself particularly agreeable to the men. One of her flirtations resulted in a disturbance at a social, two men having a fight over who should dance with her.

Her family history was as follows. The father drank a great deal though less now than formerly. Usually there were blows struck between the parents, and more than once, the patient had to run in to separate them. She always felt that her mother was jealous of her relationship with her father. As she continued treatment, the psychiatrist became identified with her husband. She was successful in keeping the treatment separate from her other activities in the hospital. However, this success was short-lived in contrast to the other patient referred to above. Since coming to hospital she had provoked her husband's jealousy by her flirtatious behaviour. Now she carried this behaviour into the transference situation. She deliberately missed an appointment and went out with a male patient instead. When she was seen two days later she was confronted with her absence, and though lying at first, she later explained exactly what had happened. She was most apologetic and asked for another chance.

During this interview, she repeated the story of her parents' quarrels, her father's frequent infidelities and her mother's jealousy. With this in mind the following interpretation of her behaviour was proposed. She had identified the doctor with her husband, and by not coming for the appointment had shown that she preferred the patient's company to his. The earlier determinant of this reaction is to be found in her identification with her father who made her mother jealous. This patient had a compulsive need to stimulate jealousy in any relationship into which she entered.

This interpretation was confirmed by the new information that the mother often accused the father of lying about his girl friends, and he would eventually confess in the same way as the patient had done. Her lies were a repetition in the present of her father's lies to her mother.

The psychotherapy described in this paper is most successful, as may be expected, with the less severe neurosis. In these cases there is no question of radical cure, but rather of a relative improvement. Improvement in this instance refers to those changes which take place while the patient remains in hospital. This improvement took place with a patient aged twenty-seven years. He was a single male who suffered from an agoraphobia of four years' standing. Altogether

he was treated for about five months, having in all about sixty therapeutic sessions. Prior to the treatment, he suffered from a degree of
tension which required four grains of phenobarbitone daily to make
life bearable. By the third month of treatment he was only taking
half a grain. The anxiety in the street became much less, although it
did not disappear completely.

In every way life was much easier for him, but it would be misleading to give the impression that he had completely thrown over
his old behaviour. In the treatment he discussed his feelings towards
his parents, his fear of sexuality and his ethical and moral values.
Throughout the time he produced very little material which could
have explained even in part, his choice of symptoms. He never mentioned anything which could have been interpreted as hostility to
the psychiatrist. It is reasonable to suppose that the improvement
could be partly attributed to the positive transference which remained undisturbed and to external circumstances.

Unfortunately there are other clinical syndromes, of very frequent
occurrence in hospitals, which do not prove amenable to psychotherapy. The first of these is the chronic traumatic neurosis. The
second is a personality defect. This defect is characterized by an
intense inhibition which extends to all spheres of activity, to work,
to the sexual life and to interests of all kinds whether physical or
intellectual. In nearly all these cases there is a suspicion of schizophrenia. They have some difficulty in thinking and communicating
their thoughts to others. Apart from this, there are never any florid
signs which would put the diagnosis of schizophrenia beyond doubt.
Some psychiatrists would call these cases schizophrenia simplex,
others schizoid personalities. These patients tend to seek admission
to a psychoneurosis hospital whereas they would hardly agree or be
considered ill enough to enter a mental hospital.

A measure of success is sometimes gained with a traumatic case
where he is allowed to talk freely and without any active interference
on the part of the psychiatrist. Once again lack of time may be the
decisive element in the apparent failure to help these patients. Improvement has occurred when the patient has seen some connection
between his symptoms and the original traumatic situation. For
example, a patient had been the victim of insomnia for some years
after his medical discharge from the Navy. His insomnia took a
peculiar form. He would fall asleep as soon as he went to bed but
wake up in a short time, and continue this waking up and falling

G

asleep throughout the night. His ship had been torpedoed at night, but he was rescued and after a short spell of leave he went back to sea. At night his anxiety was extreme, he would lie down to sleep in his clothes and do his best to prevent himself from falling asleep just in case the ship would be sunk. Usually his fatigue got the better of him and he would fall asleep. He would waken with a start in a few minutes, and then the whole cycle would repeat itself innumerable times until the morning. When he remembered all this and realized the connection his insomnia improved considerably. Instead of waking up nine or ten times in the night he would waken only two or three times.

A few improvements which occur with the traumatic neuroses do not appear with the other inhibited type of patient. Attempts are always made on a community level to adjust these patients. They require prolonged hospitalization accompanied by continuous efforts at resocialization.

At the present time a new clinical picture is more frequently appearing in hospital work. This is the psychosomatic syndrome, the peptic ulcers, the asthmatics, the hypertensives and the dermatoses. The outlook for these patients with psychiatric treatment raises the whole problem of the extent to which emotional factors are involved in their causation. If there is an emotional conflict, a frank neurosis, then the treatment is that for any neurotic illness. Only long-term therapy can decide whether the symptoms are psychogenic in origin. One patient suffering from a relatively mild hypertension accompanied by headache, dizziness, pain in the left chest and anxiety, was treated in hospital for eight months being seen every day for at least half an hour. It eventually appeared after some months that he had an associated neurosis, a mild anxiety hysteria. He did not materially improve for another six months while he was being seen twice a week as an out-patient. After eighteen months' treatment his illness was not ended. The hypertension and his physical condition remained stationary, but there was no deterioration as far as could be ascertained. The treatment of psychosomatic cases is still a research problem and it is premature for physicians, surgeons or psychiatrists to submit such patients for treatment as they would an obvious neurosis.

Mention was made above of a group of patients who do not fit into the hospital environment. These patients suffer from many different syndromes, but if rebellious behaviour or aggressiveness dominates the clinical picture there is a tendency to label the patient a 'psychopath'. These patients are certainly a trial for everyone who comes into contact with them and reactions to their behaviour on the part of the staff is understandable. For example, the woman patient who shouts abuse at the nurses or the man who refuses to conform to the hospital regulations are frequent sources of ill-feeling.

Psychotherapy has its place in the treatment of some of these cases, and all the more so when the patient's behaviour can be understood in terms of his developmental history. The question is what must the doctor's attitude be when the patient continuously infringes the hospital rules and clashes with administrators and nurses. Ideally the psychiatrist should try and show the patient the irrationality of his actions and relate it to the treatment situation where possible. In those hospitals where there is no shortage of psychiatrists, one doctor can be responsible for the patient in the administrative sense and the other act purely as a therapist. Morse and Noble (1942) give details of an arrangement of this sort.

The advice given by Chassel (1940) seems to be most applicable to our present difficulties. He does not feel, in dealing with psychotic patients, that the usual psychoanalytic policy is really very helpful to the patient who has to fend for himself throughout the day, apart from his daily session with the analyst. Although there are practically no psychotic patients in this Unit, Chassel's views are relevant to a situation where the psychiatrist must take the responsibility for his patients. The psychiatrist must accept that the patient unconsciously considers himself to be once again in the family scene and that the psychiatrist occupies the most important position in it.

A completely passive attitude on the part of the psychiatrist is meaningless to the patient unless there is an opportunity to clarify fully for him his transference relationships; to distinguish for him that which is a repetition from the past from that which is present reality. Until such opportunities become available the doctor has to realize that the patient looks to him for love, protection, restrictions, reprimands, advice and guidance, just as he has done throughout his life to those who are for him 'in loco parentis'.

The aggressive patient involves the nursing staff more acutely than any other, yet every nurse-patient relationship demonstrates how far the nurse's role in psychiatry has moved from that traditionally associated with her. This fact has been recognized by most of the psychiatrists whose work has already been mentioned. They assert that whatever the nurse's previous experience in general training, an intensive education is required particularly in psychodynamic principles. Theoretical knowledge by itself is of little value but constant discussion of cases compensates for this to some degree. The patients spend at least four-fifths of their time with the nurses, with the occupational therapists and other medical auxiliaries. Their influence on the therapeutic outcome can often be decisive.

A patient's mood and behaviour can often be traced back directly to the influence of a nurse. In the following case the nurse-patient relationship is excellently illustrated. The patient was a young man of twenty-eight years who suffered from mild obsessional and phobic symptoms. He was being treated by the type of psychotherapy described here and so an opportunity was available to observe his reactions.

At first he only alluded to this particular nurse by a memory of adolescence. He recalled that as a boy of fifteen he represented his county in an athletic contest. At the event there was a girl of his own age similarly representing the county. She wanted him to talk to her and even kept a seat free beside her at tea in the hope that he would come over to her. However, he was too shy. This was his reaction to the friendly approach of the nurse.

Later in the treatment he was able to talk about his fondness for this nurse with greater freedom. One day he expressed resentment against another male patient. At first this seemed meaningless but it subsequently appeared that this other patient used to intrude into conversation between the patient and the nurse. When this happened he would retire leaving his rival with the nurse. This was a characteristic behaviour pattern, in the face of opposition he would withdraw.

Just before this nurse was due to leave the hospital he dreamt that 'they were in love and going to be married. He took her to see his father'. His associations to the dream led away from the nurse to other girls of whom he had been fond and eventually to his mother who had died about six months previously. He had met most of these girls while serving in the Royal Air Force and he was usually posted just when his affection was growing. It was interesting to observe that his first reaction to the nurse's departure took the form of memories where he was the one who left. This was a defence against the painful thought of being left by someone he loved, just as the manifest dream reversed a sad experience into a happy one. His next reaction involved the recall of a childhood memory. When he was five years old he was often afraid his mother might go away and leave him.

At first it seemed that the nurse was mainly a substitute for his sister of whom he was very fond. Really the nurse was also a mother substitute. Many associations as well as the material described, confirmed this. This identification of the nurse and mother explained much of this attitude towards her, his shyness of talking about her and his inability to express sexual wishes for her. When the nurse left the hospital there was an exacerbation of his symptoms accompanied by depression. This was much the same reaction as when his mother died, although not as intense.

If the patient is being allowed to express himself freely in the treatment situation there is always the tendency for him to draw the nurses with whom he is in contact into the therapeutic relationship. He may confide in the nurse rather than tell the doctor or he may transfer feelings of love or hate from the psychiatrist to the nurse. Nurses must learn to distinguish which reactions are appropriate to the present situation from those which are irrational, being transferred from other situations in the patient's life. Without this appreciation the nurse will react to the patient either in an aggressive or emotional way, depending on the patient's personality and behaviour. Many nurses as well as patients are disturbed by apparently aggressive or promiscuous behaviour on the part of other individuals in the hospital. Their discomfort originates in their own unconscious difficulties which the patient's behaviour stimulates. They project the condemnation of their own guilty impulses on to the particular patient, and consequently react in an extreme way which cannot be of any therapeutic benefit.

This problem can only be dealt with adequately in those institutions where there is no shortage of nursing personnel. Bullard (1940) and others recommend that selected members of the nursing staff undergo a personal psychoanalysis. They believe that the benefit to both nurse and patient are inestimable. Although such recommendations are obviously impracticable at present, there are several which can be followed with advantage. Perhaps the most important is an educational programme for nurses utilizing the clinical material, especially those cases which can be clearly understood in the time available for treatment. This co-operative work between all sections of the medical staff encourages the interest of the nurse and prevents her from feeling that there is little for her to contribute.

Trying to understand patients' behaviour does not imply the adoption of a completely permissive attitude in the hospital. As yet there is no evidence of its therapeutic value. Simmel emphasized the need for constant vigilance against all efforts which the patient makes to repeat in action substitutes for infantile satisfactions. When a patient is being psychoanalysed this 'acting out' can be utilized in the treatment, often with benefit. Unfortunately with our psychotherapy there is no such guarantee. Even if the behaviour of patients is interpreted to them in terms of their past, the question is whether these interpretations have any dramatic significance.

A patient of thirty-four years complained of headaches and depression. While in hospital he took a great interest in the other patients, and was for ever saying that he wanted to protect their rights. He took several patients under his wing and helped them along. He said he was happier in the hospital than he had been for years. Yet he was very discontented with the treatment he was receiving. He felt the treatment did not recompense him for the effort he made to help the other less fortunate patients. He complained that he was being exhausted and was not being given the infusion of strength he required. This reproach against the doctor was similar to one he levelled against his wife.

His early childhood had been one of continuous trauma. His father died when he was very young and his mother had neglected him shamefully. It appeared that he had gone through life looking everywhere for the love he had never had from his mother. Every relationship with women had ended unhappily usually with an aggressive outburst on his part. All his object relations were based on an identification with himself. In his need to look after the other patients, in his championing of their interests, he was identifying himself with them and showing them the care which he really wanted for himself. In this situation he was in the place of his mother and the patients in his.

His stay in hospital culminated, as may have been expected in an attack of rage directed against the ward sister. He was rude and ill-mannered. Interpretations of his behaviour were of no avail. Although he recognized intellectually the connection between his behaviour in the present and his childhood reproach against his mother it did not help. As he continued in the same way he had to be discharged from the hospital.

Too often in hospital, when interpretations are made in such situations, the patient does not gain any effective insight at all—i.e. insight which will inhibit the behaviour on future occasions. When the stay in hospital is short there is no opportunity for working through the material relating to the particular action in all its many manifestations.

While short-term psychotherapy remains the only available individual psychological treatment, careful thought must be given to therapeutic aims, not in the light of presenting symptomatology but viewed from the wider aspect of personality structure. Although every neurotic symptom is at bottom a defence against deeper difficulties, there is little to be said for indiscriminately removing symptoms if these symptoms are performing a useful function in the patient's relationships with his family and work. For example, a female patient of twenty-nine years suffering from conversion hysteria was treated psychotherapeutically. Prior to her admission to hospital she had been capable of limited satisfaction in sexual relations with her husband. After seven months of treatment the symptom of which she complained had all but disappeared. In its place she found herself not only to be completely frigid but the whole sexual process was repugnant to her. This caused a great deal of unhappiness with her husband. This development, the appearance of the frigidity, would not have been amiss if treatment could have continued for another year or more. Then there was a spinster of forty-five years who suffered from hysterical visual disturbance. She was a cheerful, outgoing individual. After three to four weeks of treatment she complained of depression, a symptom she had never experienced before. The resolution of this woman's symptoms would have necessitated her realizing that her chances of fulfilling her feminine role in life were largely gone.

Such experiences drive home the conviction that if the psychiatrist is intent on symptom cure, he must be in a position either to carry out the treatment to the end or offer the patient an alternative to that of which he has been deprived.

The application of psychotherapy of this type in the present-day psychoneurosis hospital is unfortunately limited. The limitations have been touched upon above. The results with treatment extending from three to nine months are not always good even in cases with apparently good prognosis. This fact always raises the question of the worthwhileness of spending so much time on 5 per cent of the patient population. However, there is another aspect of the work which has maximal importance in the total therapeutic effort of a hospital which caters for large numbers of psychoneurotics. The cases quoted throughout illustrate how patients are influenced by the hospital *milieu* from the moment they enter the gates. The psycho-dynamic investigation of patients during psychotherapy reveals these influences at work. They can at times be demonstrated as the cause of an improvement or relapse in an individual patient. Without such therapeutic work little would be understood.

The application of the knowledge gained from the patients treated can be used, not only to understand the greater mass of patients but also to influence them in a positive direction where this is possible. One fact seems to emerge. It is that those patients do best who can develop a positive relationship with someone in the hospital struc-ture. Individual psychotherapy cannot under present circumstances measure up to the requirements of the vast numbers of psychoneuro-tic patients. It can at best act as a therapeutic agent in a small number of cases but more importantly as a guide and means of find-ing out just what happens to psychoneurotics when they come into hospital. This knowledge could not be obtained without the use of the psychoanalytic technique. We regard the Industrial Unit as a sociological and therapeutic experiment and as yet feel that we know very little about our individual patients and even less about the patient community. We do feel, however, that after careful research we are beginning to have some ideas on treatment which are not entirely intuitive. We believe that within the treatment limitations which we have to accept, very little can be done by psychotherapy alone and a wider cultural approach offers a promising field of experimentation.

REFERENCES

Breuer, J. and Freud, S. (1895), *Studies in Hysteria.*
Bullard, D. M. (1940), *Jn. Nerv. Ment. Dis.*, **10,** 70.
Chassel, J. (1940), *Psychiatry*, **3,** 181.
Fromm-Reichmann, F. (1947), *Psychoanal. Quart.*, **16,** 325.
Knight, R. P. (1945), *Amer. Jn. Psychiat.*, **101,** 777.
Menninger, K. (1940), *Bull. Menninger Clinic*, **4,** 105.
Menninger, W. C. (1936), *Amer. Jn. Psychiat.*, **93,** 347.
Menninger, W. C. (1936), *Jn. Amer. Med. Asscn.*, **106,** 756.
Menninger, W. C. (1936), *Bull. Menninger Clinic*, **1,** 35.
Morse, R. T. & Noble, D. (1942), *Psychiat. Quart.*, **16,** 578.
Rickman, J. (1948), *Jn. Ment. Sc.*, **94,** 764.
Simmel, E. (1929), *Inter. Jn. Psychoanal.*, **10,** 70.

CHAPTER VI

TECHNIQUES IN GROUP FORMATION

BY DR. B. A. POMRYN

THE difficulties of achieving any improvement in severe character disorders with short-term individual methods of treatment are all too familiar to those working in crowded out-patient clinics; in such a setting the time that can be devoted to an individual patient consists of a few minutes only at very infrequent intervals. Even in an in-patient community such as ours where the intake is controlled, a case load per doctor of twenty to thirty cases, with an average of two to three new admissions per week, makes it impossible to treat more than one or two patients by uncovering or analytic methods.

The planned routine of the Unit, which has already been described in Chapter II, provides a valuable basis for therapy, but on admission many of the patients are found to have erroneous conceptions of the aims and methods of psychiatric treatment; for example, the neurotic may express much dissatisfaction if he does not receive what he considers to be the right type of treatment. In his mind this may consist largely of seeing his own doctor for as long as possible, preferably to the exclusion of the doctor's other patients, and his actions may be largely directed towards this end. We attempt to understand the way the patient uses his environment and by explanation and interpretation achieve some improvement in his social adjustment.

Neurosis is usually accompanied by disturbance of interpersonal relationships. This may sometimes be seen more readily in a ward than in the early interviews with the psychiatrist. Thus, a patient at his first interview with the doctor appeared pleasant in manner and gave a not unfavourable impression. However, the nurses reported that in the wards he proved to be insolent and provocative; there was constant friction between himself and an older man whom he clearly saw as a model of his own father. It was known that from earliest years he had revealed an attitude of bitter animosity towards his father.

We were aware that within the spontaneous groups which emerge in the wards, some patients could be persuaded by others within these groups to perform tasks, or to refuse to perform them, more readily than in response to an individual request. It would appear that, for good or evil, a group applies social pressure to its constituent members and modifies considerably their behaviour.

In order to observe the behaviour of individual patients in a community setting all the patients allocated to one doctor were treated in one group, which for purposes of reference amongst them was termed 'Group A'. It was the routine for the Unit patients to be admitted to hospital on Mondays. For the remainder of the first week in hospital the patient was seen in individual interviews only. During this time a routine psychiatric history was recorded and a full physical examination made so that the patient could be reassured when there was no evidence of physical disease. Every patient, irrespective of his diagnosis, was then informed that beginning with his second week of in-patient treatment he would be included in a group, and that he would be expected to discuss within the group any matters which he had considered discussing with the doctor. He was informed also that apart from indications for specific physical treatments, he would not be seen alone again by the doctor before departure from hospital. It was not a common experience for patients to ask for individual interviews subsequently. Those who had to be transferred to another part of the hospital for treatment, as for example to the insulin coma ward, were encouraged to continue to attend all group meetings. Other psychiatric treatments such as modified Insulin, electrical convulsion therapy, intravenous barbiturates, or ether abreaction, were given where indicated, but this appeared to be relatively seldom. Absence from the group was discouraged, and feelings of rejection by the group avoided as far as possible. Indeed the constituent members considered it part of their function to ensure that everyone was present. If absentees were noted messengers were sent to round up the tardy ones.

Every week two or three new patients would be added to the group. An approximately equal number would be withdrawn as patients were discharged from hospital. The meetings were held four times a week in the same room in which the entire community was accustomed to meet. The total number of patients participating varied between sixteen and twenty-eight. Invariably the patients placed themselves in the fashion of a horse-shoe, facing the therapist, but with a slight gap separating them as a group from him. Nurses attended the meetings as duties permitted, and usually participated as actively as did the patients. Whenever the meagre rations permitted, a mug of tea was prepared by some of the more active members who often augmented the supply which the ward sister was able to allow, with contributions brought from their own homes.

At early meetings frequent requests were made to the leader for guidance on the choice of topic for discussion, but the responsibility for this was never accepted by him. It appeared that as the group continued a tradition gradually emerged. It was as though the longer established members came more and more to accept the group as being part of themselves and belonging to them. It became the custom for the newer patients to introduce themselves by giving an outline of their histories. Not even the most inhibited patient failed to contribute at least something of his story at his first appearance. Following this, others would develop the usual group discussion and might describe the relief frequently obtained by the free discussion of personal problems. The identification with newer members might be indicated by a remark by an older patient to the effect that emotional difficulties were possessed by all members of the group. There seemed to be value in this type of group activity, particularly as it would not be solicited by the leader. The patients indicated verbally that they considered the group to be an effective force.

The role of the leader was not an active one. He did not intrude in any of the discussions other than to correct inaccuracies, for example, fallacious physiological statements. The proceedings were kept active chiefly by a nucleus of the more intelligent and understanding patients. These tended to prevent the intrusion of what appeared to them to be irrelevant material, and they even made tentative interpretations. The average duration of a session was about one hour, when the leader would indicate that the time for ending had arrived. When, however, it was felt that the entire group was reluctant to finish the meeting, and particularly when emotions were aroused, discussions would be permitted to continue, occasionally for as long as two and a half hours. There was always a preponderance of males and at no time were there more than six females in a group. My impression was that the content of the discussion was not of prime importance. It was more the feeling that there was a body of interested people participating in something with which each individual could feel identified. Long silences did not occur and so did not constitute a problem.

Six of the most intelligent members of this large group, consisting of five males and one female, were chosen to form another relatively 'closed' group, termed 'Group B'. Meetings with these patients were held for an additional hour on four mornings a week in the same room and here the level of discussion was more intimate. It could be said that in Group A, group suggestion, persuasion and education were used, whereas in Group B a form of uncovering therapy developed and thus a greater measure of insight was achieved. Group B constituted a 'cabinet' within Group A and exerted a powerful influence inside it.

As an example of the suggestive influence of Group A, the case of a chronic hysteric is quoted. A middle-aged obese man had complained of weakness of the legs. After numerous investigations an arthrodesis had been performed on one foot some years previously; since that time he had come to exert himself less and less, and had been reduced progressively to less active posts at his place of employment. During the six months prior to admission to the Unit he had felt himself to be incapable of his last job as a gatekeeper, and was almost entirely confined to his home. He walked only a few paces at any one time and then only with the aid of a stout stick. During several group discussions it became apparent to everyone that he had grown increasingly intolerant at home and that he was tyrannizing his family. One patient suggested that perhaps the stout stick that he used functioned also as a weapon of chastisement and this indeed proved to be true. The group now indicated that they were united in believing that the patient had little physical need for the support of his stick and began to urge him to throw it away. During the remainder of this patient's stay in hospital, the stick was no longer seen, and he described his steady progress in subsequent sessions. He would proudly inform the group of unaided walks to Sutton, a distance of one mile from the ward. In addition he described an altered attitude towards his home situation and his wife confirmed this. As he thanked the group for the benefit he derived, newer members were undoubtedly impressed.

Sometimes individuals wishing to restore the desired situation of the individual interview, indicated that there was some particular tit-bit of history fitted only for the doctor's ears. The doctor would be waylaid in a corridor and an interview requested, but this was surprisingly infrequent. The patient would be told briefly that, as he had been previously informed, the group meetings were to be considered as interviews. Most patients would be persuaded to accept this and would confess in the group that there was considerable relief in relating details to a group which accepted what was told to them without censure.

It was clear that patients held the opinion that doctors' powers were mystical and that cures were sometimes akin to miracles. This belief was perhaps linked with the passive role adopted by the leader. Cures described in the popular press were cited, and one patient who had visited Lourdes was listened to avidly. At this time there was much comment in the community on the success achieved by an outside doctor using hypnosis in a case of hysterical paraplegia. It was difficult for the patients in Group A to understand why such methods could not be practised in the Industrial Unit, and on this occasion a more active role on the part of the leader was tried experimentally. One of the group was an unprepossessing, inadequate female of forty-two. Two years prior to her admission to the Unit she had been left friendless when her mother had died. She had become ill and had been treated at a mental hospital without response; she was then sent on to the Poor Law Institution, whence she had been transferred to Belmont. From the time of the death of her mother she had been unable to walk unaided. In moving from her chair to the door of the room she would get down on all fours and crawl until she reached the nearest point on the adjacent wall, would then rise to an upright position and with fingers sliding along the wall would pass rapidly to the door. An epileptic boy of twenty-four, subject to outbursts of irritability which sometimes occurred during the group meetings, had befriended her, and invariably sat beside her. He would escort her to Sutton, but in spite of his repeated exhortations, she would not walk unless given the support of his arm. It was believed that she might respond to strong suggestion and persuasion. In the presence of the entire Group A she lay on a couch and less than 0.5 mgm. of a solution of sodium amytal was injected intravenously and she was then commanded to walk. She rose, crossed the floor to the door of the room and then returned to the couch unaided. The group was deeply moved and this was alleged to be miraculous.

The apparent miracle was, however, short lived for on the following day her condition was unchanged and she informed the group that she had no recollection of having walked unaided. Although disappointment was expressed, the experience was felt to have been warranted, for the group cohesion was increased. The group decided that in addition to all efforts made on their behalf, a real desire to be well was necessary within the individual for permanent improvement to be obtained. The group redoubled its efforts to help this patient. It was interesting to note that during the treatment by persuasion just described, one patient seated by the door cried out in abject terror when the female patient approached him. He was an intelligent youngster, aged twenty-one, who had revealed his ambivalent attitude towards his father; the latter, though smaller in stature than his son, often boasted of his prowess and commented on his son's puny physique and lack of willpower in the most derogatory terms. The patient had masochistic and homosexual problems. As he was a member of Group B he discussed his terror in a meeting on the following day. He explained how he had identified the therapist with his father and felt that both had superior powers which frightened him. He had had the impression that the drugged female patient had advanced towards him during the demonstration, and that because of the condition induced by the drug, she would attempt a sexual onslaught on himself in the presence of the group.

Even severe personality disorders appear to benefit from membership of such a group. An aggressive psychopath, aged forty-four, with a criminal record dating back to childhood, was admitted to hospital because of the severity of his outbursts. In these he would smash up the home, or threaten and strike his employers on the slightest provocation. He defiantly related his criminal record to the group and boasted of his imperviousness to physical punishment. During group discussions he scoffed at the attempts of other patients to arouse his conscience. Throughout his stay in hospital nothing was seen of his aggressive outbursts, apart from a threatening attitude to an administrative clerk who, through a misunderstanding, refused to return the patient's ration book when he was due for discharge. The patient apologized verbally before he left hospital and again in writing subsequent to his discharge.

Both groups continued to function for one year. The composition of Group B remained relatively static. When a member of this group was discharged, those remaining requested the admission of a new member to maintain the original number, discussed the merits of other patients in Group A and invited one of them to join Group B. This latter group was more closely knit than Group A. At its meetings the members were seated around a circular table and there was no appreciable gap separating the leader. Patients were addressed by their christian names and the leader as 'Doc'. It was noted that the integration of this group was maintained apart from the regular meetings. The remaining patients in the community referred to them as 'the intellectuals'. Where practicable they accompanied each other in their travelling at week-ends and so aided one of their number, a female phobic anxiety case with fear of travelling, to get home each week-end. This patient had come to the group when the doctor treating her had left the hospital. He had devoted much time to seeing her individually, but she stated that she gained very much more from the group than from any other method of treatment. It appeared that the individual members of this group were loathe to give up their cohesion. Patients who had left hospital would often address letters · to the group or ask the doctor about the progress of the group. In this group a schizophrenic patient was maintained in a quiescent state for one year; another potential schizophrenic improved sufficiently to return to his studies at Oxford and having obtained a degree wrote a thesis for his M.A. degree. A very depressed man recovered his self-esteem and returned to his family which had feared that a rupture of the family structure was inevitable. Another male, the son of a doctor, had complained of depression and apathy over a period of three years. He had received an intensive course of electrical convulsion therapy, and during the twelve months prior to admission had been receiving further fits at fortnightly intervals. When he felt too much afraid to continue with them, he was admitted to hospital. He then considered that his case was hopeless, but on discharge two and a half months later he expressed deep gratitude to the group. He returned to employment and on the news of his marriage a congratulatory telegram was sent by the group to which he had belonged.

It was felt desirable to try to obtain this cohesion which seemed to lead to increased intimacy in the groups, with a number of more inhibited patients. The combination of music and drawing was introduced into the group activity. Four patients and the leader met three times a week and heard the recording of a complete classical work. Records were kindly loaned by the Arts Council of Great

Britain and augmented by a further supply from the local public library. As far as possible the items played (usually the popular symphonies, concertos and programme music) conformed with the suggestion of the group members. On one occasion dance music was played, but the patients considered this to be uninspiring and undesirable, so that this type of music was not used again. The patients were asked to draw whatever came into their minds while listening to the music. When it ceased each one described what he had drawn and was encouraged to try and indicate what the drawings implied, the others in the group commenting in any way they wished.

In another group drawing alone was used. Four patients and the doctor met for an hour two days a week; on one day the patients drew spontaneously in silence. All drawings were in pencil on ordinary typing paper. In the second weekly meeting the drawings were discussed in a manner similar to the previous group. An inadequate immature psychopath of average intelligence aged twenty-eight, drew pictures which the others thought resembled the drawings of a child. He tried to draw the faces of the other members of the group, and although there was some resemblance to the original, they all appeared as children. A depressive drew a symbolic figure which in describing he related to his present-day difficulties and to his difficulties with his parents. At the end of the hour he saw that his diagram was symbolic of an Oedipal conflict. A fetishist drew mutilated bodies and often the figures of pregnant women. He indicated that he wanted to shock the members of the group and although he could not explain why, he found that he obtained considerable easing of his tensions while drawing. An anxious male drew distortions of the human body and related this to the conceptions he had about his own body. Clearly he reflected in his drawings something of his own body image. The existence of these groups outside the meetings was never as clear as in Group B.

The use of music in the entire patient population of the Unit was next considered. A short classical extract was played at one of the regular morning meetings, and patients were asked to comment on the effects the music had on them; they were asked what they thought the music meant, or what the composer had thought of when writing the work. The tension and hostility aroused by this type of meeting was such as to lead to a rapid termination of the project.

The performance of music to a section of the community was

still, however, desirable, particularly as it was now being requested. An invitation to attend musical sessions was extended to everyone within the Unit. They were held four times a week just after lunch, during the patients' rest period. The lecture room was again used. The numbers attending varied from day to day. On Wednesday, when patients were allowed to leave the hospital for the afternoon, there might be as few as three patients, but at other times there were as many as twenty-eight patients and nurses. Here again efforts were made to obtain the requests of the patients. On Mondays only one work would be heard, and a discussion along the lines already indicated encouraged. In this group the response was much more favourable and it became possible for some individuals to present personal difficulties. On Wednesdays no attempt at discussion was made as attendances were invariably small. On Thursdays patients were handed a sheet of paper as they arrived and encouraged to draw while listening to the music. When the programme was completed each patient was asked to describe what had been drawn. Although there was no communication, identical subjects would often be drawn. Water was a very common one chosen by the patients. The Thursday meetings proved to be the best attended, although not all the patients were willing to draw spontaneously. On Fridays no discussion or drawing was suggested but several patients brought their own paper in order to draw. The music played consisted largely of the more popular works with which the patients were already familiar. Unfamiliar or long works were not easily tolerated, but some patients, particularly those who had difficulty in controlling their own aggression, delighted in hearing the recordings of modern works. The use of music continued to extend spontaneously. Patients themselves brought records into the hospital and organized recitals at which a doctor would not necessarily be present.

Patients under the care of other doctors expressed both curiosity in the functioning of groups and a desire to participate, so a group was formed to try and utilize this interest. To bring together an interested group, a meeting of all those in the Unit who wished to join in musical discussions was arranged. Nine patients and two nurses came. After hearing a piece of music the group discussed the effects on themselves. The group found this to be most interesting and requested regular meetings, so these were held once each week for an hour. Very soon, however, the group desired to discontinue

H

the music, and concentrate on discussions following the customary pattern of patient groups which they had heard about. As the constituent members were under the care of various doctors, it soon became apparent that the composition of this group would change, but it was decided to maintain the total number at eleven. When members in the room were counted the doctor was never included. This may have been because he remained completely passive and spoke only in reply to questions directed at him. When there were vacancies the remainder decided upon extending invitations to others within the community of the Unit, both patients and nurses. Most of these invitations were accepted. The composition of the group was so maintained that there were approximately equal numbers of males and females, and all types of illness were included. Many patients commented on the value of this group, and said that they wished they could have entered a group on the day of admission and so not have wasted any time. Absentees were severely criticized and it was decided to drop anyone who failed to attend two consecutive meetings. When at one time there was a preponderance of inhibited patients, silence caused increased tension. This was overcome by meeting in the dark for several sessions, on the suggestion of several patients. A man aged twenty-five, the only child of ageing parents, expressed his hostility to all those who showed any desire to help him and doubted whether anyone was sincere. He had no friends and was unemployed. He remained alone in his room except when he could obtain sufficient money to go out and get drunk. He accepted the invitation to attend this group, but sat in rigid silence refusing to answer when anyone spoke to him. Gradually, however, he came to be drawn into the group, and then to talk increasingly freely. Since discharge from hospital he attends the Unit social club at St. George's Hospital, and has made several friends.

In all that is attempted the controlling influence of the leader is of major importance to maintain the structure of the group. The goal is to achieve such a structure and obtain the maximum participation of all the members. With the bulk of patients who are apathetic and disinclined to exert themselves and perhaps display considerable hostility towards assistance offered, the first step is to encourage any form of activity. A great diversity of activities is desirable but impracticable. It is one of the most important functions of the doctor to bring this about, but the untapped resources of the patients themselves can be utilized in a community to enhance the doctor's efforts.

Social pressure as experienced in a group does seem to bring about modifications in personality even though the individual remains unaware of the mechanisms involved. Where possible interpretations have been made but in the main the handling of groups by the leader has been intuitive.

The permissive attitude adopted within a group which is largely supportive, is felt to be of fundamental importance. The leader in the above groups has adopted a largely passive role and apparently contributed little to the activities described; but the patients have always looked to him as the final authority and at times invested him with almost magical powers.

For those neurotics who believe themselves to be unique and unwanted, the group can help them to a feeling of belonging as they come to be accepted. As the group structure becomes more defined they seem to be influenced by its attitudes and accept these changes in themselves as though from inner conviction.

An important feature is the continuation of the group's work outside the organized meeting times. It has been noted that the existence of the group, particularly of Group B, could be observed within the general framework of the Unit, the constituent members choosing to remain in close proximity. Even after leaving hospital it was felt that patients desired to remain participants in a group. Thus it may have been that adjustment to a group of hospital patients was a transitional stage towards readjustment towards such groups as the family or employers and workmates.

CHAPTER VII

THE FOLLOW-UP INQUIRY—I

SOME GENERAL ASPECTS

BY JOY TUXFORD

SIX months after the first industrial case was discharged from hospital the Follow-Up Study began. Two groups were investigated; the first comprised patients who had attended the Industrial Neurosis Unit; the second was made up of disabled neurotic unemployed people who had not attended a rehabilitation treatment centre such as the Unit and who were referred to us by the employment exchanges of the Ministry of Labour. The first study was done six months after they had left hospital on 238 consecutive discharges. Of these, 104 were followed up, 19 could not be traced, 34 had been discharged for less than six months, 79 lived outside the London area, and two patients refused to be seen. The second study was made sixteen months after the first one, on 147 disabled persons. Forty-four of these could not be traced, two refused to be interviewed and 103 were visited. The object of the ex-patient follow-up was to discover how, if at all, the Unit had helped patients and, if possible, to assess to what extent group and community techniques of treatment were helping towards rehabilitation. Further, we hoped to learn what type of patient profited most from treatment in the Unit. The control study, it was hoped, would give us some basis for the comparison of a treated and an untreated group; but the difficulties inherent in matching the two groups were such as to prevent the second group from attaining the status of a fully matched control group.

The Patient Follow-Up

Upon admission to hospital Dr. Maxwell Jones took a comprehensive social record (Appendix One) from each industrial case.[1] This record comprised a detailed work history prior to the man's admission to hospital, including the length of each job, the number of years of unemployment, and the reasons why a man left each of the various jobs he had held prior to his admission, it also included details of the patient's schooling, prison and forces records, and of any previous psychiatric treatment he had received. The man was also asked to state his preference for the type of work he wanted to do upon discharge from hospital. This material was later coded and correlated with the information obtained from the follow-up study. These findings are shown in detail in Chapter VIII.

The Follow-Up Interview

Unlike the information obtained in the Social Record, which was taken as a matter of routine in hospital, the data of the follow-up record (Appendix Two) was taken in the man's home, the information being given in the course of conversation and the routine questionnaire completed after the interview.

In the main we followed Guttman's,[2] procedure and no follow-up inquiry was made by mail; each patient was visited in his own home, and thus the distortion inherent in postal surveys, was eliminated. We confined the follow-up visits to London and the Home Counties because travelling to places as far apart as Scotland and the West Country, Ireland and the Yorkshire Moors, presented a problem beyond our resources. We hoped that this sample, though not a random one, would be representative of the total group in all important respects. The figures given in Chapter VIII show that for all the available data the sample followed-up differs in only minor respects from the total group.

All visits were unannounced and no letter preceded a visit or asked for an appointment. The advantages of such a method lay in finding the man as he really was; in the kitchen, helping to bath the children or cooking the supper; in the garden, feeding the chickens or sowing cabbages; in the 'front room', studying after a day at the Government training centre; playing cards with his family, or

---

[1] For the purpose of the study an industrial case was one which, on admission to hospital, appeared to the senior psychiatrist to present a placement as well as a treatment problem.

[2] Guttman, E., *Report on Public Health and Medical Subjects*, No. 93, H.M. Stationery Office, 1946.

sometimes sharing the fireside with a glowering wife. All this could so easily be hidden if it were known that a social worker was coming, when the best china and the best manners befitting such an occasion would appear. An unannounced visit meant fruitless journeys (for 104 interviews, over 280 journeys were made); but the value of information obtained was clearly greater than would have been the case had the visit been announced and that was compensation enough for fruitless journeys and personal frustration.

The informal nature of the visit enabled us to interview the man in the family situation, where interpersonal relationships were readily apparent. In all cases the patient was encouraged to take the lead. I guided the conversation but never pushed for information. By such methods the man was seen in his home situation, coping with the interview himself, and using his family in much the same way as one would suppose he used them in other circumstances. In making qualitative assessments of the patient's adjustment since leaving hospital, and of the way he handled things, his relationships with his family served as an important guide. It also lessened the tensions, anxieties and suspicions inherent in a neurotic population of this nature when dealing with a stranger, and it increased the co-operation of the patients concerned.

In one instance I arrived at a patient's home in the midst of a family quarrel. The patient was abusing his mother, who could not accept that her son was grown up and to some extent emotionally independent of her. She had sought refuge in an hysterical illness. The father, who one felt secretly agreed with his son and was a little tired of his wife's continued invalidism, did not interfere. By the time the patient's girl-friend had arrived the battle was in full force. The son attacked his mother with a knife, the father mildly moved his chair to the edge of the group, and the girl-friend tried to remonstrate with them both. Such a situation was of considerable assistance when it came to assessing the patient's health and social adjustment, and it gave a more natural picture of the patient's interpersonal relationships than would have resulted from a more formal interview.

The purpose of my visit was, as I told each man, 'To see how you have been getting on since you left hospital.' The neurotic who loved to be the centre of attention would usually enjoy the situation, after his initial tension and anxiety had abated. Often his wife or mother was silently antagonistic or a little exasperated. She must have felt that I was encouraging the ex-patient to indulge in his symptoms and his grudges, while she, who lived with them, believed in playing them down. Silently I sympathized with her about my behaviour. After the interview, which lasted sometimes as long as three and a half hours, and never less than an hour and a half, I completed the questionnaire and the information was later coded. The detailed results of the patient follow-up are discussed in Chapter VIII.

The Disabled Person Control Study

We attempted to match our patient follow-up population with a group of untreated chronic unemployed neurotic individuals known to the Disablement Resettlement Officers (D.R.O.s) at the employment exchanges. Our aim was to compare a treated and an untreated group with similar clinical and sociological problems to see what changes, if any, had been accomplished by treatment in the Industrial Neurosis Unit. We knew that the D.R.O.s had our type of problem case to deal with, unaided, at the employment exchanges. It was not practicable for us to examine psychiatrically, possible candidates; we had to hope that, by indicating to the D.R.O.s our needs based on a preliminary analysis of our follow-up population, we would have some basis for the matching of our two groups. We attempted to match the groups as far as possible in respect of the following variables; age, marital state, service in the armed forces, education, number of jobs, wage level and clinical characteristics. We then arranged a meeting with the London Regional Office of the Ministry of Labour and discussed the number and location of the district employment exchanges which would be required to supply us with the type of material we were looking for, on the basis of a geographical analysis of the patient group actually followed-up. We next met the D.R.O.s from the relevant districts as a group, and gave them a description of the type of case we wanted. We met with some resistance at first because some D.R.O.s were anxious about their role in such a study; they were to ask those disabled men on their files whom they considered suitable for our study, if they would be willing to be visited by a social worker after a period of six months. The D.R.O.s pointed out that this was a departure from their usual relationship with their disabled persons and might stir up all kinds of anxieties. How would the disabled person interpret such a visit, no matter how carefully the nature of the inquiry had been explained to him? Would it jeopardize the relationship of the D.R.O.

with his clientele, and so on? To meet this challenge, and in order to win over the group of D.R.O.s, we resorted to a form of sociodrama with the Social Worker playing her usual role and the most anxious of the D.R.O.s impersonating his supposedly fearful disabled person. A visit of the type under discussion was acted out; once the D.R.O.s had grasped the exact nature of the inquiry contemplated, they gave us the most enthusiastic co-operation. It was decided that ten visits a month by the Psychiatric Social Worker should be aimed at. The D.R.O. was asked to select twice the required number of men, so that in the event of failure to trace men after a period of six months, we could use substitutes. More important, the D.R.O. gave us relevant data about each man and we were able to discuss clinical and other points with the D.R.O. himself, so as to obtain the best poss- ible matching with our patient follow-up population. Thus it was arranged that every month an employment exchange in an agreed sequence would select twenty men conforming to our requirements (see Appendix Three) and obtain their consent to a visit after a lapse of six months. The list was then brought to us by the D.R.O. in person for final discussions, but despite all these precautions and the extreme kindness and courtesy of the Ministry of Labour London Regional Office and the various district D.R.O.s, our control group was not strictly comparable with our patient follow-up group. It became clear soon after the control study began that the meetings with the D.R.O.s, plus the written clinical instructions as to our requirements had been an insufficient guide to help them in selection. Cases which were predominantly physical in nature were included by the D.R.O., and it was only at the time of our visit, that the true nature of the clinical problem emerged. Although the D.R.O. had done his best to meet our clinical criteria, he frequently failed, through lack of training, to differentiate between physical and psychological disability; thus cases of tuberculosis, respiratory disease, neurological problems and advanced cardiac disease would appear in the control group. Moreover, as the study continued, it became apparent that the control group was psychiatrically different from our patient follow-up group.

It is impossible in an experiment of this kind to match the two groups completely on even criteria. We placed major emphasis on clinical matching and with the limited range of choice had to forgo accuracy in varying degrees on the remaining criteria. For example the control group was significantly older than the patient follow-up group and this of course contributed to the distortion of other variables.

In view of the above findings there is no justification for giving detailed quantitative comparisons between the two groups—these might be misleading. Nevertheless the disabled person group is such an important one sociologically that some comparison between the two groups is of value.

The Disabled Person Control Interview

Since this group were completely unknown to us as individuals I originally wrote a letter asking the disabled person if I might visit him at a mutually convenient time. This approach, however, proved disappointing. Letters remained unanswered and appointments were not kept, so that I reverted to the unannounced visit similar to that used in the patient follow-up study. Even so there were some people who would not see me as, e.g. a man wanted by the police, or one who owed money to his neighbours. In such cases frequent and unannounced visits met with the same reply from tired and often harassed wives, 'I'm sorry, but he's out, call next Monday and he'll be in'. In a group of 147 men approached, two consistently refused in this way.

The technique of this interview was different from that of the patient follow-up. I could not inquire here, as with the earlier group, how the individual had fared since leaving hospital. Instead I told him something of the research and what we hoped to achieve by it. This explanation satisfied most people, although there were some who were rather paranoid and saw the survey as a campaign by the Government to ascertain the 'goings on' of each citizen. Such people proved very difficult to interview, and the picture obtained from the visit was naturally distorted. In all cases, however, the home visit was preferable to an interview at the labour exchange or at a psychiatric clinic. However much a man might distort his answers, he could not completely alter his interpersonal relationships as seen in the home.

With the disabled persons group I always made use of the questionnaire. I had come for information and therefore I had to record it. If I failed to do so the disabled person often became suspicious. Unlike the patient group, where the interview revolved around the patient, the interview now revolved around me. I was in charge of the situation and guided the conversation, dispensing with the questionnaire as soon as was practicable.

In this control study I took a record of the man's employment, health and social activities for the six months prior to my visit, and also an account of his activities since leaving school; this gave us information comparable to that which we had got from our patients during the first week of their stay in hospital.

Some General Impressions of the Disabled Persons Control Study

The group of disabled persons appeared to be in part a mixture of people similar to the ones we admit to hospital, with a large percentage of psychotics who should have been in a mental hospital. The remainder were disgruntled people who presented hopeless employment problems and who appeared to be past seeking, or benefiting from, any help that could be given to them. In addition there were those whose complaint was mainly a physical one.

As has been mentioned earlier, the age of the disabled person group was significantly higher than that of the patient group. Three times as many disabled persons as patients were unemployed for the period of six months prior to the follow-up visit. According to the social worker's assessment approximately the same number of people in both groups were suitable for sheltered employment, and for employment on the open market but under sheltered conditions. However, nearly twice as many patients as disabled persons were thought to be capable of normal employment, while twice as many disabled persons as patients were classified as unemployable.

In both groups, 50 per cent of those people in employment at the time of the visit had held only one job during the six months prior to the follow-up visit, though the average length of total unemployment was much higher in the disabled person group.

At the time of the follow-up, the wage of the patient group tended to be higher than that of the disabled person group, and showed an increase on their average wage prior to admission.

According to the P.S.W.'s assessment of health, the ex-patients tended to be in better health than the disabled persons; four times as many disabled persons as patients were assessed as having very poor health, while three times as many patients as disabled persons were assessed as being in good health. It is interesting to note that the majority of patients were optimistic about their future health, while the majority of disabled persons were pessimistic.

The majority in both groups had had no treatment in the six months prior to the visit, while the next largest group had visited their panel doctor. Significantly fewer ex-patients than disabled persons had attended the out-patient department of a general hospital. The ex-patient group made a significantly better social adjustment than did the disabled person group.

There is a very similar distribution of figures for both groups as to type of household. By far the largest groups in both studies were living in unsatisfactory or fair households.[1]

There is detectable throughout an interesting attitude to the Ministry of Labour. The ex-patients, whether they were doing well or badly, did not project their frustrations on to the Ministry of Labour or the D.R.O.s to the extent that the disabled persons did. During the control study of disabled persons it became clear to me that the job of the D.R.O. was an extremely difficult one, especially with regard to those embittered and disgruntled neurotics who had been unemployed for a very long period. These people were not sufficiently disabled to warrant admission to hospital and had either not thought of, or resisted, the idea of psychiatric help.

I was impressed by several things in the course of both studies. It was interesting to find such a diversity of cultures within the London area. Hackney as a group was as different from Ilford as Barnsley is from Edinburgh. In each area different values were accepted and different mores found. The responsibility assumed by the family varied in different areas of London. In Ilford, and other outer suburbs such as Hillingdon and Ealing, the family tended to accept much responsibility for the patient's illness, trying to do what they could for him. In other areas, however, such as West Ham and Hackney, where overcrowding was more prevalent and caring for the sick comparatively difficult, illness became the concern of officials and Ministries. In some parts of London illness was most definitely a community affair, the responsibility being borne by the group and not by the family as it was elsewhere.

The disabled person group had a much weaker sense of 'belonging' to a group than had the patients. The stay in the Unit was so much more for the patient than a period in which he saw his doctor at regular intervals and received treatment. During his stay he was incorporated into a community which had its own culture, its own way of looking at problems, and its own way of dealing with them. In the morning meetings the patient learnt about his body and about

---

[1] The meaning attached to the descriptive term 'fair and reasonable' is discussed in Chapter VIII.

his emotions, as well as his symptoms; more important, the Unit gave him, sometimes for the first time in his life, a place in society. He ceased to be an isolated individual and became a functioning member of society, dependent upon other members and with a real responsibility towards them. This more socialized outlook had remained with most patients six months after their discharge from hospital.

The member of the disabled person control group had rarely belonged to any closely integrated group. He may have been to a mental hospital, or to a Government training centre, but more often he had sought help from his general practitioner or the out-patient department of his local hospital. He knew he was an employment problem, 'a nuisance' (to quote many of them) 'to the D.R.O. and the Ministry of Labour who can do little for me'. In addition he may have been a victim of a mental disease which frightened him and his family, and which was little relieved by a weekly visit to his doctor. Only one man expressed whole-hearted belief in the doctors, and few had belief in anything. The patients had a specific attitude towards unemployment and neurosis, and a way of dealing with both problems, which appeared not to have deserted them six months after discharge from hospital. The disabled person in comparison had much less to rely on. Often I was left with the impression that the disabled person felt rejected by society, not only on account of his employment difficulties, but also because of his neurosis.

In both groups there was an interesting attitude to unemployment. Neither group showed any guilt about their unemployment. They expected to be without work at some time or another because of their disability, and being registered as disabled persons with the Ministry of Labour seemed to foster this attitude. However, in some cases where unemployment itself aroused no guilt it seemed that a neurotic illness did, and for this reason the man wanted to work in order to distract attention from his illness.

Throughout the study I was impressed by the paucity of community life. The family, which was in most instances a small and loosely-knit group, was often the only one which had any real meaning for the individual. The 'community', which was only a vague concept to these men, could not give much needed support. Too often the individual was thrown on his own quite inadequate resources to solve problems of an emotional nature.

It became increasingly obvious, as I proceeded with the follow-up, that the patients had an immense advantage in having the services of the two hospital D.R.O.s at their disposal. Most of the disabled persons interviewed had found their own jobs, with often poor results, and collectively they had little faith in the D.R.O. or the Ministry of Labour. Where our D.R.O.s placed a man, however, the probability of a good subsequent adjustment was high.

Nearly all the disabled persons asked for help at the interview. They wanted a job, or treatment, or both. In most cases the Ministry of Labour was felt to be of little or no help. Pills and medicines, with an occasional visit to an out-patient department, no longer held out very much hope. As a group they had little faith in anything. This led me to realize that compared with the ex-patient group the disabled persons lacked much which the patients had received in hospital and which had apparently helped them to make a good adjustment after discharge from hospital.

Both Follow-Up Studies had an amusing as well as at times a frustrating side. Travelling in London by public transport was often difficult, and long walks through lonely dockside streets or dark suburbs were bewildering and sometimes frightening.

The happiest visits were to those patients who were doing well. They were often proud of their achievements and grateful for the help they had received while in hospital. Besides the ones who had done well, even those patients who had been less fortunate and made a mess of things generally welcomed a visit and in many cases asked for help. From a contact with the hospital a man who was sick or encountering employment difficulties often seemed to gain new heart to plan again as he had been encouraged and taught to plan while in hospital. The more difficult visits, the ones that needed greater reassurance and more careful handling, were those where the patient was struggling along just managing to cope but wondering how long he could continue. Here Belmont loomed rather ominously, I felt; in such cases the visit may have done some harm, except that, should the worst happen and the man lose his job or have a relapse, a contact had been made.

In the course of my visiting I have been mistaken for the football pools representative, and real disappointment has followed the revelation of my true identity; instead of giving the patient and his family several thousand pounds which would have made an end of bad housing, poverty, and insecurity, I have asked them to give me information. I have also been mistaken for the tally man who comes at regular intervals to collect money from those people who belong to a clothing club. Only with great difficulty did I get an audience here. I have interviewed people in kitchens, backyards and on door-steps and in one-room homes, the dirt and squalor of which is difficult to believe.

In conclusion, it seemed to me personally from the rather cursory experience I gained of the community structure in all parts of London that there was in most areas a real paucity of group life; mainly due, I felt, to the fact that in many cases there was no real geographical cohesion and no focal point on which the inhabitants could centre their emotions. In addition, there appeared to be no social cohesion from within the group. Problems which arise within a group or small community are nowadays solved outside the group. The juvenile delinquent, who is a product of a certain group which to some extent bears the responsibility for his delinquency, is helped by the Probation Officer, who in all cases stands outside the group unit. The irate husband and wife who need someone to settle their differences, likewise make recourse to the Courts. The problem of poverty, of educating and maintaining children, are in nearly all cases dealt with by officers who are often not an integral part of the community from which the specific problem has arisen.

With the lessening of individual responsibility of one member in a group to another plus the increased responsibility of the State in the functioning of the normal family, there has been a decline in the individual awareness of the role required of each group member and their relationships to one another. This has led to disintegration of the group and thereby the support given by the group to the individual has in part disappeared.

The experience of the Unit has shown the prime importance of the group to the individual, both in hospital and during the often difficult period of readjustment after treatment is at an end.

It would seem that healthy groups do help to make healthy individuals, and that to ensure within a community, however small, the proper functioning of group life is to do much to provide an environment in which people can hope to lead a full life.

APPENDICES TO CHAPTER VII

APPENDIX ONE

INDUSTRIAL NEUROSIS UNIT (Research 1)
EMPLOYMENT RECORD

Name   *Age*   *Hospital No.*

Admitted   *Discharged*
Intelligence

---

1. *Method of referral.*

---

2. Date of onset of present illness.
3. Weight below optimum (on admission).
4. Registered as disabled person?   (Date)
5. *EDUCATION*

| *Type of School* | *Standard reached* | *Top Standard* | *School Leaving Age* | *Schools* |

Interruptions   (Frequent change of school or illness).

Higher Education or University.

---

6. Delinquency (Civil or Military).

7. *FORCES RECORD*

   (*a*) Date of enlistment.
   (*b*) Date of discharge.
   (*c*) Rank attained.
   (*d*) Nature of work.
   (*e*) Courses.
   (*f*) Trade tests.
   (*g*) Invalided (? Neurosis).
   (*h*) Pensions (amount).
   (*i*) Was pension for neurosis?
   (*j*) P.o.W.

8. OCCUPATION
   Type of Work   Period   Salary   Reason Leaving   Date

9. *Type of Work by Skill* (tick off)
   (a) Professional and managerial.
   (b) Minor executive posts.
   (c) Skilled workers (training period of three years).
   (d) Semi-skilled (training period two weeks to three months to two years).
   (e) Unskilled dextrous (training period two weeks to three months).
   (f) Unskilled ordinary (no training).
   (g) Casual work.

10. *Type of Work by Exertion*   (tick off)
    (a) Heavy frequent (50 lb. or more frequently).
    (b) Heavy occasional (65 lb. or more occasionally).
    (c) Moderate frequent (25 lb. to 49 lb.).
    (d) Moderate occasional (35 lb. to 64 lb.).
    (e) Light non-sedentary (up to 24 lb.).
    (f) Light sedentary.

11. Total number of jobs.   (a) Before service.   (b) After service.
12. Longest single employment.
13. Total unemployed time.
14. Total length of unemployment, prior to admission to hospital.
15. Nature of previous psychiatric treatment (give date).
    (a) Hospital.
    (b) Out-patient.
    (c) G.P. or M.O.
    (d) None.

16. Employment goal (on admission)
    (a) Return to last job.
    (b) Different job with same firm.
    (c) Wants another job (nature unknown).
    (d) Wants another job (nature known).
    (e) Starts specific training.
    (f) No interest in any job.
17. Employment difficulties (patient's opinion).
18. Main cause of nervous breakdown (patient's assessment).
19. Number of accidents.
20. Whether a trade union member or not.

21. Do you think you are in the occupation you are best suited for?
22. Have you ever been?
23. If No to the above then what do you think you are best suited for?

DOCTOR'S EVALUATION OF EMPLOYMENT PROSPECTS ON ADMISSION

24. Unemployable.
25. Sheltered employment.
26. Normal employment.
27. General impression of employment prospects.

APPENDIX TWO

P.S.W. Follow-Up Work Sheet

1. Name.
2. Address.
3. Home circumstances (lodgings, living with in-laws, etc.)
4. Informant (patient and/or relative).
5. Registered as disabled person (date).
6. Has pension been altered since leaving hospital?
7. Patient's attitude to pension.
8. Patient's attitude to Ministry of Labour.
9. Patient's attitude to emigration.
10. Patient's attitude to doctors (psychiatry).

WORK RECORD

11. Occupation since leaving hospital.
    (a) Type of work.
    (b) Hours of work.
    (c) Dates.
    (d) Salary.
    (e) Reasons for leaving.
    (f) Absenteeism (giving reasons).
    (g) Travelling difficulties.
12. Total unemployment since leaving hospital.
13. Period between leaving hospital and starting work.
14. Was first job on leaving hospital, decided on in hospital?
15. If so what part did psychiatrist play in choice?
16. If so what part did psychologist play in choice?
17. If so what part did hospital D.R.O. play in choice?
18. If so what part did local D.R.O. play in choice?
19. Any other factors determining choice.

20. What determined each choice subsequent to the first one (through employment exchange, friends, etc.)?
21. Has work been satisfactory? (Specify which jobs.)
22. If not, specify factors making work unsatisfactory (separate answers for each job).
23. Social factors at work (present employment).
    (a) Relations with employer.
    (b) Relations with fellow-workers.
    (c) Relations with foreman or immediate superior.
    (d) Any other social difficulties (working with women, too crowded, too isolated, etc.).
24. Was 'green card' or 'neurotic record' a handicap? (Specify each instance giving full factual information.)
25. Was 'green card' or 'neurotic record' a help? (Specify each instance.)
26. Does patient know if he was taken on under the Quota Scheme? (Specify instance.)
27. Does patient know what Quota Scheme means?
28. Does he think that the Disabled Persons Employment Act really helps him?
29. If patient went to a G.T.C. was he satisfied with the training?
30. Had he any placement difficulties following completion of training?
31. Comments on work record by relatives.
32. Employer's or foreman's comments on work record.
33. Does patient think he has the most suitable job that he can reasonably expect under present circumstances?
34. If not then what in his opinion would represent a more suitable job?
35. P.S.W.'s assessment of patient's present value on labour market (employment on open market, sheltered employment, or unemployable).

HEALTH RECORD

36. List of present symptoms, if any.
37. Does patient feel in normal state of health?
38. Present state of health with that on discharge from hospital.
    (a) Better.
    (b) Worse.
    (c) Same.
39. If relapsed then length of time the patient remained well after leaving hospital.
40. If still unwell, are there any new contributory factors since leaving hospital?
41. Does his job contribute to his present state of ill-health, if any?
42. Re-admission to hospital. (Type of hospital and details of treatment received.)
43. Attendance at a psychiatric out-patient department. (Number of attendances, type of treatment, etc.)
44. Visited by P.S.W.
45. Attendances at panel doctor's surgery (frequency, cause, etc.)
46. Physical treatment not apparently related to neurosis (for example, intercurrent pneumonia).
47. Any accidents at work since leaving hospital?
48. If improved or recovered during hospital treatment what was improvement contributed to?

49. Suggestions as to how the hospital treatment and general routine could be improved to assist the recovery of other patients.
50. Patient's attitude towards possible future ill health.
51. P.S.W.'s assessment of present state of patient's health.

SOCIAL RECORD

52. Does subject feel that satisfactory social adjustment has been achieved?
53. Has social adjustment been better, worse, or unchanged since leaving hospital? (Details.)
54. If unsatisfactory social adjustment give reason—at home, at work, at leisure?
55. Composition of family.
56. Housing conditions.
    (a) Physical (too small, bomb damage, etc.).
    (b) Social (in-laws, overcrowding, etc.).
57. Financial worries.
58. Patient's gross income (salary plus pensions and/or allowances).
59. Other family income (wage-earners, family allowances, etc.).
60. Leisure pursuits (games, clubs, pubs, dog racing, etc.) and percentage of time in each.
61. Leisure spent alone or in company.
62. Does patient feel that he was happier socially in hospital than at present?
63. Any evidence of anti-social behaviour.
64. Any contact with ex-Belmont patients.
65. Informant's response to P.S.W.'s visit.
66. P.S.W.'s assessment of patient's social adjustment.

APPENDIX THREE

Belmont Hospital . . . . Industrial Unit.
Control Group Recruited from Local Employment Offices

We need an adult neurotic population with the following characteristics. They must have an obvious neurosis and represent a placement problem. In the main they should be men known to you, because of their difficult personalities and tendency to complain. People who appear to be over-whelmed by their difficulties which seem to preoccupy them to the exclusion of most other topics. They seem to show little energy or initiative in finding new work. A small fraction of the whole (two or three in each batch of twenty) should be obviously too ill to work—e.g. depressed, obsessional, fainting attacks or obviously 'queer', and in these cases your attentions will be focused primarily on their mental state which to you seem to make them unemployable.

1. Age ....

2. Married or single ....

3. Forces record ....

4. Education ....

5. Number of jobs since 1946 ....

6. Income last job ....

7. General remarks ....

Note: The preliminary distributions had previously been made available to the D.R.O.s concerned.

CHAPTER VIII

THE FOLLOW-UP INQUIRY—II

*STATISTICAL ANALYSIS AND THE CONCEPT OF
GENERAL ADJUSTMENT*

BY JOSEPH SANDLER

I

THE patients of the Industrial Neurosis Unit of Belmont
Hospital are distinguished from most other neurotic groups
by the fact that they have been selected as patients on the basis
of specific disturbances of working capacity, over and above any
other manifestations of neurotic illness or character disorder. It is the
therapeutic aim of the Unit to modify the patient's behaviour so that
he will be better fitted to cope with the problems that beset him in
real life; and in particular the Unit aims at improving his capacity in
the sphere of work. The techniques used in this connection have been
described elsewhere in this volume and need not be elaborated here.
But any evaluation of these techniques and of the effect of the Unit
as a whole on each individual patient, can only be undertaken in the
light of factual knowledge of what happens to the patient after his
discharge from hospital. How well in fact, do the Unit's patients
adjust to their environment after leaving hospital? And what distinguishes those patients who do well from those who make a poor
adjustment?

An attempt has been made to answer these two important
questions by the follow-up carried out on the Unit's patients and
described in the previous chapter. In addition an experimental follow-
up study has been made on a comparative group which has not
passed through the Industrial Unit, in order to obtain data which
might throw some light on the functioning of the Unit. This second
follow-up group and the techniques used in its study have been

described, and as a discussion of this group is not relevant to the present material its further consideration will be left until later.

The visit paid by the Psychiatric Social Worker to those industrial cases which were followed up, elicited a mass of information which included data bearing on the patient's adjustment in different spheres. The term 'adjustment' is used here to indicate the degree to which the patient has successfully coped with the demands of reality; successfully that is, by the conventional standards of Western society. Adjustment may be measured in a number of different behavioural areas, and in a number of ways in each area. Thus adjustment in the work situation might be measured by such things as the wage being earned at the time of the P.S.W.'s visit, or by the number of days the patient has worked in the period following his discharge. Which of these, we may ask, should be taken as the index of adjustment in the work field? The first is in a way a measure of the patient's work adjustment at the time of the visit, while the second takes into account one aspect of his behaviour during the whole six months following discharge from hospital. Both are measures of adjustment in relation to work, and yet neither comes near to describing the complete adaptation made by the patient in this sphere.

Ideally, all the possible different adjustment measures should be used, but this is prevented by the practical difficulty of having to answer the question 'How well has the patient done?', by reference to a multitude of measures. The tracing of the relationship between the data collected in relation to the different patients while they were in hospital, to all these adjustment measures, would be a task which, if not impossible, would be sufficient to dishearten the most enthusiastic statistician.

There is, however, a possible way of overcoming the difficulties inherent in the use of a large number of indices of adjustment. This is by attempting to reduce the number of measures so that *what is common* to a representative set of adjustment measures is taken as the essence of adjustment. Those measures of adjustment which seem to cover the different aspects of the field under investigation can be reduced in such a way to their common denominators, and these common denominators may be used as the yardstick against which we assess the recovery of our patients.

The practical method of seeking these common elements is some form of factor analysis, and such a method was applied to eleven measures of adjustment derived from the data collected by the P.S.W. in her follow-up interview. These eleven criteria were chosen from the point of view of the expressed therapeutic aims of the Unit, and converted into quantitative scales.

Explanations of the basis of assessment are given below.[1]

(I) *P.S.W.'s assessment of patient's health*

		Cases
Very Good	(all-round improvement—no symptoms)	5
Good	(coping well with symptoms)	19
Fair	(managing to cope adequately)	39
Poor	(needs treatment—symptoms influence whole life)	24
Very Poor	(badly needs treatment or should be in hospital)	5
No Information		2

(II) *P.S.W.'s assessment of the patient's value on the labour market*

	Cases
Employable on open market	43
Employable on open market under sheltered conditions ... (sympathetic employer and ideal conditions of work)	26
Employable under sheltered conditions	13
Unemployable	12

(III) *Total unemployment in last six months*

	Cases
Nil	46
1 week	9
2–6 weeks	7
7–11 weeks	9
12–16 weeks	5
17–21 weeks	1
22–26 weeks	17

[1] The final distribution of results (which comprise a larger number of cases than used in the determination of the general adjustment factor) is given for the first five items as these are later referred to in the text. In addition to the ninety-four patients listed for these five items, ten patients were found on follow-up, to be in mental hospitals or in prison.

(IV)   *Wage at time of P.S.W.'s visit*

	Cases
£2 per week or less	5
£3 ,, ,,	8
£4 ,, ,,	11
£5 ,, ,,	21
£6 ,, ,,	15
£7 ,, ,,	5
£8 ,, ,,	2
£10 and over	3
Unknown	1
Unemployed	23

(Keep was taken as £2 10s. to £3 per week according to type of keep. Tips and food were taken as £2).

(V)   *P.S.W.'s assessment of social adjustment*

		Cases
Very Good	(very satisfactory—many social activities)	6
Good	(coping well, has outside interests)	32
Fair	(apathetic but some interests)	32
Poor	(few interests, very apathetic)	15
Very Poor	(unsatisfactory—no social interests)	8
No Information		1

(VI)   *Average length of job in past six months*
Totally unemployed patients were given a score of 0.

(VII)   *Patient's assessment of improvement since leaving hospital*
Better, worse, or the same since discharge.

(VIII)   *Social adjustment at work*
Very good (gets on well with everyone).
Good (gets on well with most).
Fair (gets on not too badly with others, but keeps mostly to himself).
Poor (suspicious of most—is not liked).
Very poor (hates all others at work).

(IX)   *Average wage in last six months:* The totally unemployed group were given a wage of 0. (Average wage while working only.)

(X) *P.S.W.'s estimate of standard of environmental conditions*
No account was taken of suitability.
Very good—good dwelling and furniture—comfortable.
Good—reasonable conditions.
Fair—conditions not too good—badly furnished.
Poor—very poorly furnished—very limited accommodation.
Very poor—unfit to live in—Rowton House.

(XI) *Proportion of working time at work*
The negative of absenteeism. Patient's own estimate. Unemployed group received 0 for this item.

At the time that the statistical analysis was started, results were available for eighty-two patients. Using these results, the matrix of product-moment intercorrelations between these measures was computed, and factored by Thurstone's Centroid Method.[1] This yielded a most gratifying result. The correlations could almost completely be accounted for by one common general factor which contributed 41.3 per cent of the variance of the original measures. The saturation of each measure with this common quality is given below.[1]

	Saturation
P.S.W.'s assessment of the patient's health	0.853
P.S.W.'s assessment of the patient's value on the labour market	0.833
Number of days employed in six months	0.802
Wage at the time of P.S.W.'s visit	0.793
P.S.W.'s estimate of the patient's social adjustment	0.786
Average length of job in last six months	0.705
Patient's assessment of improvement in his health	0.649
Social adjustment at work	0.396
Average wage in last six months	0.277
P.S.W.'s estimate of standard of environmental conditions	0.255
Proportion of working time at work	0.108

[1] 41.3 per cent of the variance of the eleven measures accounted for by the general factor is high in this field. Even in the analysis of intelligence tests, where factor-analytical techniques have yielded their best results, the amount of variance accounted for by common factors is often of this order of magnitude.

The factor saturations are in effect the correlations of the adjustment measures with the single common factor, and it will be seen that five are above 0.75. It is certain that three of the four lowest saturated measures— viz. social adjustment at work, average wage in last six months, and proportion of working time at work (the negative of absenteeism) suffered an increased unreliability owing to a number of distortion effects. The common factor accounts for 66.3 per cent of the variance of the five highest measures.

The results of the factor analysis indicate that it is legitimate to speak of the patient's *general adjustment* after his discharge from the Unit, for this single factor common to all the measures is manifestly a general tendency to make a good or bad 'adjustment'. It is a synthesis of eleven different measures of adjustment, and is their common core.

At this point it might be well to mention the possibility of so-called 'halo-effect'—i.e. the tendency for the ratings and assessments to be influenced by the rater's general impression of the individual rated. Almost certainly the assessments are not completely free from its influence, and indeed it must enter into all subjective ratings. If it does enter to any considerable extent, it must be regarded as a limitation to the accuracy of the original measurements, but it does not invalidate the use of the general adjustment factor as the best measure of the common elements in the description of the patient as he appeared at the follow-up interview. Against the possibility of strong influence of halo effect we must weigh the fact that the P.S.W. was on her guard against it, and the fact that the relatively objective measures such as number of days employed in six months and the wage at the time of visit, have extremely high saturations with the general factor.

The investigation of the relation between general adjustment and all the antecedent data[1] was now a practical possibility. The regression equation for general adjustment was calculated, enabling an 'adjustment score' to be computed for each patient. Patients who were in prison, or in mental hospitals after six months, were given a score of 0. The distribution of these scores for the 104 patients followed up is given in Fig. 1. The mean adjustment score for these patients is 8.24 with a standard deviation of 4.57.

A patient's position on the scale of general adjustment enables one to say how he has succeeded in relation to other patients, but in itself

[1] Information recorded in hospital—work record, test results, diagnosis, etc.

it gives no indication of how well patients have adjusted by conventional social standards. Nevertheless we may gain an idea of the meaning of a high or low adjustment by reference to the individual measures of which the adjustment score is a composite. Thus the

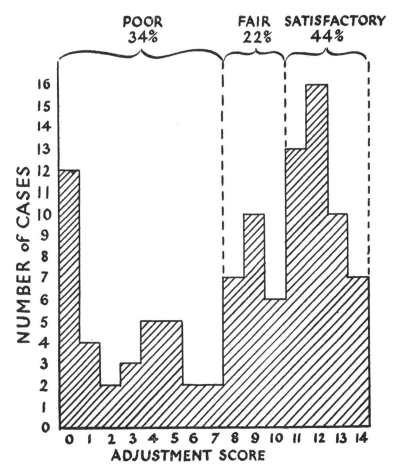

Fig. 1.—The distribution of adjustment scores for 104 patients.

P.S.W., in her careful estimate of the patient's mental health, placed 61 per cent in the 'good' 'very good', and 'fair' classes. Similarly, her estimate of their value on the labour market showed that 41 per cent of the patients were considered employable on the open market, while a further 25 per cent were considered employable on the open market but under sheltered conditions. The (cautious) estimate of social adjustment made by the P.S.W. showed 37 per cent having made a good or very good social adjustment, while 67 per cent had made a fair social adjustment or better.

The more objective measures fully support these figures. The distribution of the number of days employed during the six-month period shows that 53 per cent were employed for at least twenty-five weeks in the twenty-six week period. Forty-four per cent had a wage at time of visit of £5 per week or more, while 55 per cent earned £4 or more.

On the basis of these results we may put forward with a fair degree of confidence the statement that those with an adjustment score of 11 or more have made a satisfactory adjustment (44 per cent). In addition we may say that those having adjustment scores of 8 to 10 have made a 'fair' adjustment or better. The dividing lines are shown in Fig. 1, but it should be borne in mind that they are to a large extent arbitrary.

II

In this section some account will be given of the way in which patients distribute themselves in each of the items assembled under the heading 'antecedent data', such data being available for 237 patients in all. Admission numbers of the patients dealt with range from 1 to 248, but of those who were given admission numbers, 11, for a number of reasons did not stay long enough for a work record to be taken. The single exception was the second patient admitted to the Unit, who was followed up before the decision to exclude this group was made. This patient is included in the 104 follow-ups, but as no antecedent data were recorded for him, he is not included in the group of 237 patients, and the follow-up group in this section contains 103 patients. The mean adjustment score of the group followed up, excluding this one patient, who obtained an adjustment score of 1, is 8.31.

The grouping of the patients after discharge is summarized as follows:

	Cases
Living outside London	79
Discharged less than six months before the analysis of data began	34
Not traced	19
Followed up	103
Refused to see P.S.W.	2
Total	237

In the tables given below, the headings T.G. (total group), F.U.G. (follow-up group), and M.A.S. (mean adjustment score) will be used. The 103 patients listed under F.U.G. are included under T.G.

For each item, the frequency distribution of the members of the follow-up group in the categories composing the item was tested statistically either by *chi-square* or *Student's t* to see if it was significantly different from the distribution of those patients not followed up. The level of statistical significance adopted was 5 per cent, and it was found that for the great majority of items, the differences in the distributions of those followed up and those not followed up was attributable to chance. For those few items where the difference in frequency distribution is significant, possible reasons for the difference are given, and unless any mention is made to the contrary, it may be taken that the follow-up group is representative for the item under discussion.

The mean adjustment scores for patients falling into the various categories for each item of the antecedent information, have been tested for statistical significance, in most cases by analysis of variance, the level of significance adopted being 5 per cent.[1] If there is a significant association between any item and adjustment score, the item might quite feasibly be used for the purpose of predicting later adjustments. Where a correlation is quoted, it is non-linear and derived from the analysis of variance unless otherwise stated.

In Section III of this chapter, implications of the statistical results will be discussed.

---

[1] Because of the non-normal distribution of adjustment scores, the tests used are not strictly applicable. However, they give some indication of the significance level and their predictive power should be tested by further research.

1.	Age on admission	T.G.	F.U.G.	M.A.S.
	16–20 years	18	6	8.8
	21–25 ,,	59	29	8.3
	26–30 ,,	58	24	7.9
	31–35 ,,	45	17	9.4
	36–40 ,,	19	8	9.7
	41–45 ,,	18	7	6.6
	46–50 ,,	13	8	6.4
	51–55 ,,	5	2	12.0
	56–60 ,,	2	2	6.5

The mean age of the follow-up group is 31 years, which is also the mean age of those not followed up. The standard deviation of age for the F.U.G. is 8.9 years, and for the remainder of the patients 9.5 years.

The differences in M.A.S. are not statistically significant, and we may conclude that there is no significant relation between age and adjustment.

2.	Sex	T.G.	F.U.G.	M.A.S.
	Male	216	94	8.2
	Female	21	9	9.1

Initially a number of female patients were included, but after a short while only male patients were classed as industrial cases. The difference in adjustment between the two sexes is insignificant.

3.	Admission Number	T.G.	F.U.G.	M.A.S.
	1– 20	17	14	7.3
	21– 40	20	14	6.1
	41– 60	19	12	8.3
	61– 80	20	10	8.5
	81–100	19	9	6.6
	101–120	19	7	11.1
	121–140	20	9	9.7
	141–160	19	5	10.2
	161–180	19	5	12.4
	181–200	20	6	7.0
	201–220	19	6	7.0
	221 +	26	6	10.7

The admission number is an indication of the point in the life of the

Unit at which any patient was admitted. All industrial cases were numbered, although a number left within the first two days and were not included in the total group.

The group followed up is not representative of the total group in respect of time of admission to the Unit. This difference is statistically significant at the 1 per cent level, and may be accounted for by the fact that the earlier admissions tended to be from the London area, and it was only after the Unit became more widely known that a larger proportion of admissions came from more distant areas. Those who lived out of London were not followed up, and thus the F.U.G. contains a significantly higher proportion of the earlier admissions.

The product-moment correlation between admission number and adjustment score is 0.200 which is significant at the 5 per cent level. Later admissions to the Unit have done significantly better six months after discharge than the earlier admissions.

4.	*Length of stay in the Unit*	*T.G.*	*F.U.G.*	*M.A.S.*
	1– 30 days	36	15	5.3
	31– 60 ,,	67	24	9.2
	61– 90 ,,	58	32	8.5
	91–120 ,,	33	17	8.5
	121–150 ,,	16	6	10.0
	151–180 ,,	9	3	6.0
	181–210 ,,	9	5	10.8
	211–240 ,,	4	0	—
	241–270 ,,	3	1	8.0
	271–300 ,,	1	0	—
	301 + ,,	1	0	—

The mean length of stay of the total group is 80 days, with a standard deviation of 56.8 days. The F.U.G. has a mean stay of 78 days and a standard deviation of 48.5 days. The difference in mean length of stay between the follow-up group and the rest of the patients is not statistically significant.

Those who have stayed a month or less in the Unit have the lowest M.A.S. and this is possibly due to the influence of four patients who were discharged within a month of admission and sent to mental hospitals. As the figures stand, the differences in the M.A.S. are not statistically significant.

5. *Registration as a disabled person*

The majority of industrial cases had been registered as disabled persons at some time before their admission to the Unit.

	T.G.	F.U.G.	M.A.S.
Registered as disabled before admission to hospital	141	61	8.2
Not registered	96	42	8.5

There is no significant relation between registration as a disabled person before admission, and adjustment subsequent to discharge.

6. *Mode of referral*	T.G.	F.U.G.	M.A.S.
Ministry of Pensions	52	20	8.7
Out-patient Departments	131	66	8.5
National Association for Mental Health	5	2	5.5
Ministry of Labour	23	8	6.4
Ex-Service Societies	15	2	6.0
Belmont Hospital	1	0	—
Mental Hospitals	5	3	8.0
Other sources	5	2	11.0

The particular source through which patients have been referred to the Unit bears no significant relation to subsequent adjustment.

7. *Time from onset of illness to admission to Unit*	T.G.	F.U.G.	M.A.S.
Less than 6 months	8	6	11.2
6 to 11 months	19	9	9.8
1 year to 1 year 11 months	39	19	10.2
2 years to 2 years 11 months	32	11	7.6
3 years to 3 years 11 months	29	10	7.8
4 years to 4 years 11 months	16	5	5.6
5 years to 5 years 11 months	20	7	6.9
6 years to 6 years 11 months	19	7	3.9
7 years to 7 years 11 months	12	7	8.9
8 years or more	36	18	7.9
Gradual	6	4	9.5
Unknown	1	0	—

If the four 'gradual' cases are omitted, the product-moment correlation between the length of time from onset of illness and adjustment is –0.233, which is significant at the 2 per cent level for ninety-nine cases, and is in the expected direction. Length of illness at the time of admission is significantly associated with a poor adjustment after discharge.

8.	Marital Status	T.G.	F.U.G.	M.A.S.
	Single	140	59	7.5
	Married	88	40	9.5
	Widowed	4	2	4.5
	Divorced	0	0	—
	Separated	5	2	13.5
	Other	0	0	—

The M.A.S. for single and married men are significantly different at the 5 per cent level. This indicates that married persons do significantly better after discharge than those who are single.

9.	Wage in last job before admission	T.G.	F.U.G.	M.A.S.
	£1–£1 19s. 11d.	6	2	12.0
	£2–£2 19s. 11d.	8	4	12.0
	£3–£3 19s. 11d.	18	11	6.1
	£4–£4 19s. 11d.	45	20	8.9
	£5–£5 19s. 11d.	42	19	8.7
	£6–£6 19s. 11d.	18	5	11.8
	£7–£7 19s. 11d.	7	5	10.2
	£8–£8 19s. 11d.	4	3	11.0
	£9–£9 19s. 11d.	1	0	—
	£10 +	2	1	5
	Not known or no work since demobilization	86	33	6.8

It was decided, for this and other wage items, to test the difference in M.A.S. between those for whom a wage is given, taken as a single group, and those for whom the wage is unknown or who have held no job since demobilization. The difference is significant at the 2 per cent level, and corresponds to a correlation of 0.230.

The differences in M.A.S. at the different wage levels is not statistically significant.

10. *Highest wage in any job*

	T.G.	F.U.G.	M.A.S.
£1–£1 19s. 11d.	1	0	—
£2–£2 19s. 11d.	8	3	11.7
£3–£3 19s. 11d.	19	10	7.9
£4–£4 19s. 11d.	24	14	6.1
£5–£5 19s. 11d.	48	21	9.8
£6–£6 19s. 11d.	31	11	9.7
£7–£7 19s. 11d.	21	11	9.6
£8–£8 19s. 11d.	10	6	6.8
£9–£9 19s. 11d.	4	0	—
£10 +	17	11	8.7
Not known	54	16	6.3

The difference between the adjustment of those for whom the wage is given, and those for whom the wage is not known, just fails to be significant, and corresponds to a correlation of 0.190.

For those for whom a wage is given, there is no significant association between the recorded highest wage and adjustment.

11. *Average Wage*

This referred to the period after discharge from the Forces, or for those not in the Forces, to the period from May 1945. Periods of unemployment have not been taken into account, and the average wage was arrived at by a simple averaging of the different wages earned by each patient.

	T.G.	F.U.G.	M.A.S.
£1–£1 19s. 11d.	8	2	13.0
£2–£2 19s. 11d.	8	4	8.0
£3–£3 19s. 11d.	15	9	9.0
£4–£4 19s. 11d.	52	22	8.0
£5–£5 19s. 11d.	37	13	10.9
£6–£6 19s. 11d.	13	6	10.0
£7–£7 19s. 11d.	6	5	6.6
£8–£8 19s. 11d.	2	1	12.0
£9–£9 19s. 11d.	2	0	—
£10 +	2	1	13.0
Not known	92	40	7.0

The difference between the M.A.S. of the 'not known' group, and the remaining patients taken as a single group, is significant at the 5 per cent level and corresponds to a correlation of 0.210.

The difference in the M.A.S. of the different wage levels is not statistically significant.

12. *Type of work (skill)*
This refers to the last job held by the patient before admission.

	T.G.	F.U.G.	M.A.S.
Professional and managerial	1	1	0.0
Skilled (training three years or more)	20	12	10.8
Semi-skilled (training 3–35 months)	97	48	8.0
Unskilled dextrous	46	16	9.0
Unskilled ordinary	62	22	7.9
Casual work	10	4	6.3
Unspecified	1	0	—

The relation between type of work (skill) and adjustment after discharge is not statistically significant.

13. *Type of work (exertion)*
This also refers to the patient's last job.

	T.G.	F.U.G.	M.A.S.
Heavy frequent (50 lb. or more frequently)	6	3	5.3
Heavy occasional (65 lb. or more occasionally)	5	2	10.5
Moderate frequent	28	13	7.9
Moderate occasional (35–64 lb.)	111	45	8.0
Light non-sedentary	65	28	9.7
Light sedentary	21	12	7.0
Unknown	1	0	—

The differences in the M.A.S. are not statistically significant.

14. *Longest single employment*

	T.G.	F.U.G.	M.A.S.
Less than 1 year	10	4	10.8
1 year	42	15	6.7
2 years	39	20	7.2
3 years	39	23	9.0
4 years	24	7	8.3
5 years	20	8	10.8
6 years	12	6	7.7
7 years	7	3	9.0
8 years	6	3	10.7
9 years or more	36	14	7.9
Not known	2	0	—

There is no significant relation between the length of the longest period of employment, and subsequent adjustment.

15. *Unemployment time immediately prior to admission*

	T.G.	F.U.G.	M.A.S.
Nil	50	18	9.9
One month or less	39	19	8.9
2 to 3 months	41	19	7.1
4 to 6 months	26	9	11.0
7 to 9 months	20	8	7.1
10 to 12 months	13	7	8.6
13 to 18 months	16	7	7.1
19 to 24 months	14	9	8.4
2 to 3 years	8	4	5.0
More than 3 years	7	3	3.7
Not known	3	0	—

The product-moment correlation between unemployment time immediately prior to admission and adjustment is 0.163. This is not statistically significant, unless we take into account that it is in the expected direction, in which case it would just be significant at the 5 per cent level.

16. *Total unemployment time*

	T.G.	F.U.G.	M.A.S.
Nil	16	8	10.5
Less than 3 months	32	13	9.1
4 to 6 months	24	8	10.6

	T.G.	F.U.G.	M.A.S.
7 to 9 months	13	8	9.0
10 to 12 months	30	13	5.5
13 to 18 months	31	12	8.2
19 to 24 months	27	13	9.4
2 years 1 month to 3 years	31	12	7.8
3 years 1 month to 6 years	18	8	4.3
6 years 1 month to 10 years	6	3	9.7
More than 10 years	3	1	13.0
Not known	6	4	9.3

There is no significant relation between total unemployment time before admission to the Unit, and adjustment after discharge.

17. *Previous psychiatric treatment*	T.G.	F.U.G.	M.A.S.
No previous psychiatric treatment	30	12	10.8
Out-patient treatment or visits to G.P.	69	32	7.7
In-patient treatment	138	59	8.2

The differences in the M.A.S. for the different categories are not significant as they stand, but if the group of patients who have had no treatment is compared with those who have had some sort of treatment, the difference in the M.A.S. is significant at the 5 per cent level, and corresponds to a correlation of 0.197.

18. *Education*	T.G.	F.U.G.	M.A.S.
Elementary	163	67	8.5
Secondary	25	9	8.1
Technical schooling	9	8	7.4
Higher education (including university)	19	8	6.1
School certificate or matriculation	6	3	7.0
Boarding school	4	2	11.0
Private school	3	2	10.5
Other	6	3	9.0
Less than two years school	1	0	—
Not known	1	1	13.0

The differences in educational level are not significantly associated with adjustment after discharge from the Unit.

19.	Scholarship	T.G.	F.U.G.	M.A.S.
	Scholarship gained in school	27	12	8.4
	No scholarship	210	91	8.3

The gaining of a scholarship while at school is unrelated to adjustment after discharge from the Unit.

20.	Record of juvenile delinquency	T.G.	F.U.G.	M.A.S.
	Yes	17	4	7.8
	No record	220	99	8.3

The differences in the M.A.S. are not statistically significant.

21.	Breaks in schooling	T.G.	F.U.G.	M.A.S.
	No breaks in schooling or serious illness during school years	185	80	8.0
	Break in schooling or disturbed schooling through illness	52	23	9.3

The difference in the M.A.S. is not statistically significant.

22.	Adult offences	T.G.	F.U.G.	M.A.S.
	No record	205	91	8.5
	Some offence	32	12	7.3

The difference in the M.A.S. is not statistically significant.

23.	Trade Union membership	T.G.	F.U.G.	M.A.S.
	Not at any time	159	74	8.3
	At some time but not at time of admission	36	14	8.7
	Member of a trade union	38	14	8.4
	Not known	4	1	0.0

The differences in the M.A.S. are not statistically significant.

24.	Suitability of last job	T.G.	F.U.G.	M.A.S.
	No job has been suitable	113	50	9.5
	Suitable	33	18	7.1
	Does not know	8	4	12.5
	Has been in suitable job but not last one	83	31	6.6

This refers to the last job held by the patient before admission to the Unit, and is the patient's own estimate of its suitability. The differences in the M.A.S. are statistically significant at the 1 per cent level, and correspond to a correlation of 0.314.

25.	Accident proneness	T.G.	F.U.G.	M.A.S.
	Not prone to accidents	191	82	8.3
	Prone to accidents (2 or more accidents at work)	43	19	8.8
	Not known	3	2	4.5

This was estimated by the P.S.W. from the patient's account of accidents he may have had. It is not significantly related to subsequent adjustment.

26.	Family history	T.G.	F.U.G.	M.A.S.
	Unknown	38	17	7.6
	Negative	99	39	8.6
	Positive for siblings but not parents	11	4	4.5
	Positive for other relatives	3	0	—
	Parents had psychotic breakdown	12	8	7.4
	Parents had neurotic breakdown or were psychopathic	21	12	7.4
	Parents had neurotic personality	51	23	9.8
	Other	2	0	—

The differences in the M.A.S. are not statistically significant.

27.	Primary cause of breakdown	T.G.	F.U.G.	M.A.S.
	None or unknown	48	21	8.8
	Domestic or social difficulties	32	17	9.1

	T.G.	F.U.G.	M.A.S.
War strain or experience	33	16	7.7
Job unsatisfactory	3	2	4.5
Accident	23	8	9.1
Gradual or many causes	10	2	2.0
P.o.W. stress	14	6	8.2
Other causes	21	11	11.0
Forces training	29	11	6.9
Somatic disorder	24	9	6.8

This was the patient's own opinion of the primary cause of his breakdown. It is not significantly related to subsequent adjustment.

28. *Pension*

	T.G.	F.U.G.	M.A.S.
Not in Forces	61	31	8.2
No pension at any time	93	42	7.9
Pension since ceased	6	3	11.7
In receipt of pension	77	27	8.7

The differences in the M.A.S. are not statistically significant.

29. *Employment difficulties (patient's estimate)*

	T.G.	F.U.G.	M.A.S.
None or unknown	23	8	7.6
Mainly nervous illness	81	40	7.5
Mainly physical illness	19	7	8.6
Own personality	26	11	7.2
General ill-health (mental and physical)	38	17	8.3
Other reasons	50	20	10.8

The differences in the M.A.S. are not statistically significant.

30. *School-leaving age*

	T.G.	F.U.G.	M.A.S.
10 years old or less	1	0	—
11 years old	1	0	—
12 years old	0	0	—
13 years old	8	3	4.7
14 years old	168	71	8.4
15 years old	20	9	11.7
16 years old	23	11	6.6
17 years old	9	6	8.2
18 years old	7	3	6.3

The differences in the M.A.S. are not statistically significant.

31.	Employment goal	T.G.	F.U.G.	M.A.S.
	No interest in future jobs	12	3	9.7
	Wants to return to last job	21	11	6.8
	Wants a different job with the same firm	3	1	9.0
	Wants another job (nature known)	102	47	8.6
	Wants another job (nature unknown)	85	35	8.0
	Wants to start a specific type of training	11	4	9.5
	Would take any job	3	2	11.0

This was the goal expressed by the patient. The differences in the M.A.S. are not statistically significant.

32.	Prisoner-of-war	T.G.	F.U.G.	M.A.S.
	Not a P.o.W.	211	90	8.2.
	P.o.W.	26	13	9.4

The difference in the M.A.S. for the two groups is not statistically significant.

33. *Total number of jobs since leaving school*
This applies to those who have not been in the Services. Those who have been in the Forces are dealt with in items 34 and 35.

	T.G.	F.U.G.	M.A.S.
In Services	176	72	8.4
1 to 5 jobs	20	11	10.0
6 to 10 jobs	17	7	10.4
11 to 15 jobs	8	5	6.2
16 to 20 jobs	3	3	4.0
21 to 30 jobs	5	3	5.3
31 to 40 jobs	1	0	—
41 to 50 jobs	3	1	11.0
Not known	4	1	1.0

For the thirty cases for whom the total number of jobs is available the correlation with general adjustment is 0.268. This is not statistically significant.

34. *Total number of jobs before service in Forces*

	T.G.	F.U.G.	M.A.S.
No service	61	31	8.2
No jobs	9	2	12.0
1 job	21	8	7.6
2 to 3 jobs	64	22	9.6
4 to 5 jobs	37	16	7.6
6 to 7 jobs	19	9	9.4
8 to 9 jobs	8	3	6.3
10 to 11 jobs	3	2	9.0
12 to 14 jobs	3	0	—
15 to 17 jobs	5	4	6.8
More than 17 jobs	9	5	6.6
Not known	1	1	3.0

The differences in the M.A.S. are not statistically significant.

35. *Total number of jobs since service in Forces*

	T.G.	F.U.G.	M.A.S.
No service	61	31	8.2
No jobs since service	24	9	7.4
1 job	32	12	10.7
2 to 3 jobs	42	19	8.7
4 to 5 jobs	29	10	9.3
6 to 7 jobs	20	7	8.7
8 to 9 jobs	11	5	5.0
10 to 11 jobs	4	2	7.0
12 to 14 jobs	3	2	4.5
15 to 17 jobs	1	0	—
18 or more jobs	6	4	6.0
Not known	4	2	8.5

The differences in the M.A.S. are not statistically significant.

36.	*Invalided out of the Forces*	T.G.	F.U.G.	M.A.S.
	Not in the Forces	61	31	8.2
	In Forces, not invalided	45	23	8.5
	Invalided, not neurosis	33	17	9.6
	Invalided with neurosis	98	32	7.6

The differences in the M.A.S. are not statistically significant.

37.	*Rank held in Forces*	T.G.	F.U.G.	M.A.S.
	Not in the Forces	61	31	8.2
	Private or equivalent rank	131	58	8.0
	N.C.O. or officer	45	14	10.1

The differences in the M.A.S. are not statistically significant.

38.	*Courses attended in Forces*	T.G.	F.U.G.	M.A.S.
	Not in Services	61	31	8.2
	Battle training	11	6	6.2
	Trade courses	51	22	9.6
	General educational courses	3	0	—
	Other	1	0	—
	None	109	44	8.1
	Not known	1	0	—

The differences in the M.A.S. are not statistically significant

39.	*Trade tests taken in Forces*	T.G.	F.U.G.	M.A.S.
	Not in Services	61	31	8.2
	Not taken	151	59	8.5
	Tests taken	24	13	7.8
	Not known	1	0	—

The differences in the M.A.S. are not statistically significant.

40.	*Length of service in Forces*	T.G.	F.U.G.	M.A.S.
	No service	61	31	8.2
	1 to 12 months	19	9	7.7
	13 to 24 months	19	12	10.4
	25 to 36 months	20	7	7.0
	37 to 48 months	20	6	7.8

	T.G.	F.U.G.	M.A.S.
49 to 60 months	21	7	7.9
61 to 72 months	24	16	8.3
72 months +	22	8	10.5
Regular Army	31	7	5.9

The F.U.G. is not representative of the total group, the difference being statistically significant at the 2 per cent level. This is mainly due to the greater tendency for those who have had service in the Regular Army, to come from outside London.

The differences in the M.A.S. are not statistically significant.

41. *Diagnosis*	T.G.	F.U.G.	M.A.S.
Predominantly depressive state	18	9	11.0
Anxiety features predominant	41	21	9.8 .
Hysterical features predominant	38	21	9.2
Aggressive psychopath	13	5	7.6
Inadequate psychopath	56	23	6.8
Organic (including epilepsy)	20	5	8.0
Schizoid character—schizophrenia	29	11	5.5
Paranoid character	3	2	11.5
Obsessional features predominant	9	2	9.5
Other diagnosis	5	1	7.0
Undetermined	5	3	4.3

Diagnosis is significantly related to adjustment six months after discharge, at the 5 per cent level of statistical significance. The association corresponds to a correlation of 0.302.

42. *Preliminary psychiatric assessment*

On the day of admission, each patient was seen for a short while by the senior psychiatrist, who made a prediction of the man's employability after treatment at the Unit.

	T.G.	F.U.G.	M.A.S.
Unemployable	22	9	4.8
Sheltered employment	40	15	6.3
Normal employment	154	73	9.2
Impossible to say	21	6	7.8

The association between the preliminary assessment and subsequent adjustment is significant at the 1 per cent level of statistical significance. This corresponds to a correlation of 0.291.

43. *Main treatment received*

	T.G.	F.U.G.	M.A.S.
No specific treatment	21	11	4.2
Small groups	27	10	9.8
No regular therapy through interview	114	53	7.9
Modified insulin	8	4	8.3
E.C.T.	1	0	—
Regular psychotherapy through individual interviews	63	25	10.5

The differences in the M.A.S. are statistically significant below the 1 per cent level, and correspond to a correlation of 0.356.

44. *Weight below optimum value*
This was assessed by the patient himself.

	T.G.	F.U.G.	M.A.S.
Weight not below optimum	125	54	8.1
Weight below optimum	107	49	8.5
Not known	5	0	—

The difference in the M.A.S. is not statistically significant.

45. *Attendance at workshops*

	T.G.	F.U.G.	M.A.S.
Not gone to workshop	53	27	6.3
Other occupation in hospital	65	33	8.9
Hairdressing	11	3	10.3
Tailoring	21	6	7.5
Plastering	25	6	10.0
Bricklaying	23	6	12.0
Carpentry	38	22	8.5
More than two shops	1	0	—

The workshops were not fully established until some little while after the foundation of the Unit. For this reason a proportion of the patients did not attend workshops, and a fair number occupied themselves with some other occupation in hospital. The workshops had comparatively few of the patients who had passed through the Unit at the time the analysis of the data began.

The follow-up group is not quite representative of the total group, the difference between the F.U.G. and the rest of the patients being significant at the 2 per cent level. This is in fact due to the greater degree of attendance at the workshops of the more recent admissions to the Unit, who had not been followed up as they were discharged less than six months before the analysis of the data began.

The differences in the M.A.S. are significant at the 5 per cent level of statistical significance. This corresponds to a correlation of 0.251.

46. Success in workshops or other training

This is the instructor's general estimate of the patient's success in the shop, taking into account both his ability and adjustment to shop conditions.

	T.G.	F.U.G.	M.A.S.
Not attended workshops, nor any other occupation	53	27	6.3
Excellent	9	3	11.3
Good	50	26	9.1
Average	50	17	10.4
Poor	27	12	5.8
Work is unsuitable	21	8	9.6
No report given	27	10	9.4

The differences in the M.A.S. are statistically significant at the 1 per cent level of statistical significance. This corresponds to a correlation between this item and adjustment after discharge from the Unit of 0.344.

47. Nurse's report

This referred to the patient's co-operation in the wards, and was coded in retrospect, i.e. in many cases some time had elapsed between the departure of the patient, and the nurse's assessment of his co-operation with other patients and staff on the ward.

	T.G.	F.U.G.	M.A.S.
Unobtainable or doubtful	99	52	7.2
Good	55	21	10.5
Average	42	16	10.3
Poor	33	11	6.5
Good at times, at other times bad	8	3	8.3

The differences in the M.A.S. are statistically significant at the 1 per cent level, and correspond to a correlation of 0.309 with general adjustment.

The difference in the M.A.S. of those patients whose behaviour the nurses could not recollect, or were doubtful, and those patients for whom a rating is available, is statistically significant at the 1 per cent level.

48. *General improvement in hospital*

	T.G.	F.U.G.	M.A.S.
No change or cannot say	74	23	4.2
Slightly better	115	53	9.3
Very much better	42	23	11.7
Slightly worse	2	0	—
Very much worse	4	4	0.0

This rating of general improvement in hospital was made by each patient's doctor on the rating scale shown above. The differences in the M.A.S. for the different 'improvement' groups is highly significant. The variance ratio F is 28.27 for 3 and 99 degrees of freedom. This corresponds to a correlation of 0.667 between improvement in hospital, and adjustment in the six months after discharge.

Psychological tests

The results of these will be dealt with in the chapter on vocational guidance.

III

The data in Section II of this chapter serve two main functions. First, the distributions of cases for the various items give an idea of the make-up of the Unit population, and are given in some detail to facilitate comparison with other populations. Secondly, they indicate the relation between some of the antecedent measures and general adjustment in the six-month period following discharge from the Unit.

The fact that a number of antecedent measures are significantly related to adjustment means that it is possible to predict which patients will do well, and which badly, to a degree of accuracy better than might be expected by chance alone. It is clear that as these results apply to one particular type of population, they should only be applied to other groups with great caution, but it is believed that they afford a basis for the pre-selection of those cases which will profit from treatment of the type given in the Industrial Unit. This problem of prediction will be discussed further in the chapter on Vocational Guidance. Some of the implications of the results shown in Section II will be discussed below. The material will be divided into two parts. First, those items of information will be discussed which were recorded by the senior psychiatrist at his intitial interview, and are relatively objective in that they consist of replies to a standardized set of queries. Secondly, the psychiatric and other assessments made during the patient's stay will be considered.

Initial interview

No significant relation has been found between age (item 1) and adjustment. It appears that the older patient with neurotic employment difficulties, is on the average, likely to do as well as the younger patient. It is possible that this is the outcome of two factors operating in opposite directions. The first is that older patients may have resisted breakdown for many years, but give way finally under severe stress. The second factor is that the younger patients are less resistant to modifying influences such as we believe operate in the Industrial Unit. It may of course be that neither of these factors operate, and the capacity to effect an adjustment is quite unconnected with age in this type of patient, but this seems a more doubtful hypothesis than the former.

Admission number (item 3) is significantly related to general adjustment, a result which indicates that later admissions to the Unit have done significantly better than those admitted earlier. The general impression gained by all members of the Unit staff is that there has been no detectable change in the quality of the patients admitted, and it would seem that the better adjustment of later admissions is due to an increase in the effectiveness of the whole Unit. The general impression throughout has been that the most important therapeutic factor has been the growth of a sustained group culture, which belongs to the Unit over and above any single group of patients. This will be referred to again at the end of this chapter, where some suggestions to account for the therapeutic effect of the Unit are put forward.

Length of stay (item 4) does not correlate significantly with adjustment, which means that there is not sufficient evidence to discard the hypothesis that there is no relation between the two measures. This may also be due to the effect of two contradictory tendencies. Patients who do well quickly, and are easily placed, will tend to be discharged earlier. But severely ill patients, who develop symptoms which make it impossible for them to be treated in the Unit, will tend to be discharged earlier too.

Mode of referral (item 6) does not correlate with subsequent adjustment, which suggests that patients from the two main sources, viz. hospital out-patient departments and the Ministry of Pensions, do not differ at all in their capacity for adjustment.

That married patients do significantly better than patients who are single (item 8) is a result which might be explained in a number of ways. It would seem probable that married men have a better capacity for adjustment to begin with, as the attempt to establish some sort of marital relationships indicates at least an initial attempt to establish adult social relations. But perhaps as important, married men often benefit from the support that comes from being a member of a family group, even if this group only consists of two members.

Registration as a disabled person (item 5), trade union membership (item 23), and the receipt of a pension of any sort (item 28), do not relate significantly to adjustment after discharge from the Unit. Rather surprisingly, the length of the longest single employment (item 14), and total unemployment time (item 16) do not show any significant association with adjustment, though one may suspect that the situation is complicated by the operation of many other factors.

The three items dealing with total number of jobs before admission to the Unit (items 33, 34, 35), show no significant relation to adjustment. This result is consistent with the finding that patients of different ages do as well, on the average, after discharge.[1] The type of work involved in the patient's last job, whether graded by skill (item 12) or by exertion (item 13), does not predict at all his adjustment after discharge.

Certain features of the patient's work record are significantly associated with general adjustment after discharge from the Unit. Length of unemployment immediately prior to admission (item 15) correlates significantly with lack of adjustment, if we take into

[1] Total number of jobs correlates—0.268 with adjustment, but the number of cases (thirty) is not sufficient for it to be taken as statistically significant.

account the fact that the correlation is in the theoretically-expected direction. This result closely relates to that found for the length of illness at the time of admission to hospital (item 7), which is significantly associated with adjustment. The finding is not unexpected, as chronicity of illness has always been taken as indicating a poorer prognosis.

One of the most interesting findings is the fact that the answer to the question 'was your last job suitable?' significantly discriminates between those who did well and those who did badly after discharge. Those who considered their last job suitable, or who considered that they had at some time been in a suitable job, do significantly *worse* than those who were of the opinion that no job had been suitable. The reason for this difference lies perhaps, not in the finding of a suitable job for those who had never had one, but in the attitude of those patients whose orientation was towards their own neurotic symptoms *per se*, and not towards social and employment difficulties. Many of these patients were preoccupied with their own particular neurotic symptoms, and the Unit emphasis on social readjustment was perhaps lost to them.

In the three items that refer to wages (items 9, 10, and 11), it appears that while the different wages reported do not significantly predict subsequent adjustment, the fact that a patient can give exact details of his wages received, is significantly associated with adjustment, in two of the three items. In the third (item 10), the difference between 'known' and 'not known' just fails to be significant, unless we take account of the fact that it is in the expected direction, in which case it is statistically significant at the 5 per cent level. The patient who cannot remember the wages he has earned, or is doubtful about his information, tends to do less well after discharge from the Unit. This links up with the suggestion made to account for the significant difference in adjustment for the answers to the question on the suitability of previous jobs. Lack of interest in the details of past jobs significantly indicates a poorer adjustment.

A history of accident proneness (item 25) does not mean anything in respect of later adjustment, nor does the fact of being under weight on admission (item 44).

Family history (item 26) is not significantly associated with adjustment. It is possible that a positive family history would be associated with neurotic breakdown in the general population, but in this case we are dealing with a specially selected population. The

Unit group consists of patients who have broken down, especially in the sphere of employment, and it seems that once this has happened, a positive family history is not important in the prediction of adjustment after treatment.

The patient's statements of his employment difficulties (item 29), of the primary cause of his breakdown (item 27), and of his employment goal (item 31), do not significantly relate to his adjustment. The attitude expressed by patients in the first few days of their stay may change radically with continued discussion with other patients in the group meetings, and after talks with their doctor. It is clear that the patient's idea of the cause of his breakdown, and the cause of his employment problems, may be far removed from the real causes, and that his particular choice of 'reasons' does not predict his adjustment after discharge from the Unit.

Only 13 per cent of the patients admitted to the Unit have had no previous psychiatric treatment (item 17), and this fact testifies to the general severity of the neurotic difficulties of the Unit patients. Those who have had no previous psychiatric treatment, in spite of their small number, do significantly better after discharge than those who have had some form of previous treatment. This result is to be expected, for on the whole those patients who have failed to profit from other forms of treatment will tend to be more resistant to the Unit's influences. Nevertheless, a good proportion of those who have had previous psychiatric treatment fall into the 'good' or 'fair' adjustment groups.

Type and standard of education (item 18), or the winning of a scholarship at school (item 19), are not significantly related to adjustment. Similarly, school-leaving age (item 30), and breaks in schooling (item 21) are unrelated to adjustment.

Neither a record of juvenile offences (item 20), nor adult convictions (item 22), are significantly related to adjustment in this group. It is clear that the factors which create employment difficulties are operating within each patient, and if he manages to overcome his work difficulties, he will be able to make a good adjustment, in spite of a record of criminal or civil offences. Moreover, the structure and culture of the Unit is such, that a record of previous offences does not place a patient outside the group; many patients who were social outcasts before they entered the Unit, were able to become integral members of the patient community.

A number of items deal with record in the Services (items 32, 37,

38, 39, 40) and their relation to adjustment is uniformly statistically insignificant.

Psychiatric assessments and other ratings made in hospital

On entering the Unit, each patient has a brief interview with the senior psychiatrist. At the end of this interview, a prediction is made of the patient's employability after discharge from the Unit (item 42). This is significantly associated with adjustment after discharge, the relation being equivalent to a correlation of 0.291. It follows that a single short psychiatric interview will enable a better-than-chance selection of patients to be made, but it seems clear that any pre-selection of patients can be assisted if certain items of information obtained by the P.S.W. are used to supplement the initial psychiatric interview.

The doctor's diagnosis (item 41) is made at some time during the patient's stay at the Unit, and the crude diagnostic categories into which patients were forced for the benefit of the statistical analysis are significantly related to subsequent adjustment. It appears therefore, that although diagnoses have different meaning for different doctors, there is some central core of agreement which has a statistically significant prognostic value, corresponding to a correlation of 0.302.

More valuable than either of the two items discussed above in the prediction of adjustment, is the type of treatment afforded by his doctor to each patient. The relation with adjustment corresponds to a correlation of 0.356. If the doctor decides to treat his patient by regular individual interviews, or by small groups, then the patient will make a significantly better-than-average adjustment after discharge. It is difficult to say whether this effect should be attributed to the therapeutic effect of individual interviews and small groups, or to the selection by the doctor for more intensive treatment of those patients who would benefit from treatment. It is probable that both factors operate though their relative weight cannot be stated.

The fact of attendance at one of the workshops (item 45) significantly predicts adjustment, equivalent to a correlation of 0.251, while instructor's assessment of general success at the occupation (item 46) was even more predictive of general adjustment after discharge, the correlation being 0.344. These two items will be discussed in greater detail in the chapter on Vocational Guidance.

The relation of the nurse's report (item 47) to subsequent adjustment is interesting. The different categories significantly predict adjustment, equal to a correlation of 0.309. Those patients who are 'good', i.e. co-operative and pleasant in the ward, have the highest adjustment score after discharge (10.5), while those who are rated 'poor' have the lowest adjustment score (6.5). The heavy burdens of the nursing staff often occasioned some delay in obtaining an assessment, and it is more than statistically significant that those patients for whom a rating was unobtainable or doubtful, on the whole made a worse-than-average adjustment after discharge (7.2).

The most striking result of all has been found in the connection between the doctors' assessments of improvement in hospital (item 48), and general adjustment in the six months after discharge. This significant relation is equivalent to a correlation of 0.667, which is unusually high for this type of data. Assessments of the degree of improvement were made by the various doctors who have worked on the Unit, who would presumably employ different criteria in their evaluation of the same case. Psychiatrists' ratings are notoriously unreliable (statistically), and it is certain that were correction made for the unreliability of the assessments, even this high correlation would be substantially raised.

The assessment of improvement is made at the end of the patient's stay, and is based on two main types of criteria. The first is purely clinical, and refers to improvement in the neurotic symptoms complained of by the patient. The second set of criteria relate to change in the patient's attitude and ability to work, and to change in his capacity for social adjustment, as shown by his behaviour in the Unit. It should be stressed that this measure refers to *change* while in the Industrial Unit, for patients vary in the depth and severity of their illness on admission, although they all have employment difficulties.

The importance of this result should not be under-estimated, for it implies that the schizophrenic or severe neurotic who improves slightly during his stay has in general, a better capacity for general adjustment after discharge than the apparently mild neurotic with employment difficulties, who shows no change. In actual fact, such cases were by no means uncommon.

From the statistical results and from the subjective impressions of the Unit's staff, it seems clear that the efficiency of the Unit has increased with time. We have constantly been aware that this is a function of the accumulation of a certain set of traditions and habits

—in short, of a group culture, peculiar to the Industrial Neurosis Unit at Belmont Hospital. This growth of tradition is clearly seen in relation to the psychodrama, but similar traditions have grown up in connection with every other activity on the Unit. In the beginning the Unit was a collection of individuals, of patients and staff. Gradually it has become much more than this. The growth of a group culture meant that a certain set of beliefs and habits were taken over by each patient on entering the Unit. The existence of this culture made it possible for each patient to develop an initial identification with the group, to become part of the Unit by adopting the habits and traditions that were common to all its members, and which have been described elsewhere in this volume. Some patients absorb the group culture well, others to a lesser degree, and it seems probable that it is the degree to which this initial identification can take place, irrespective of the severity of the patient's illness, which determines his accessibility to the Unit's influence. Even manifestly hostile patients can identify themselves with the whole group to some degree, and this, we believe, opens the door to improvement.

This identification with the Unit group means the acceptance of the ideas and attitudes expressed in and by the group of patients and staff, although such acceptance may often be largely unconscious. The constant discussion of problems, and the learning of new social techniques (e.g. dancing), together with the support derived from being a member of the Unit, all have an ego-strengthening effect. In a way, the culture of the whole group is absorbed into each individual patient (introjected), and appears to stay with many as a strengthening framework to their personalities, for at least six months after leaving hospital. The degree to which the culture of the Unit is absorbed, is probably reflected by the degree of improvement during the period in the Unit.

CHAPTER IX

VOCATIONAL GUIDANCE

BY JOSEPH SANDLER

IN this chapter I should like to describe the routine of vocational guidance in the Industrial Unit; to comment on the efficiency of these procedures, and to put forward certain views on the problem of vocational guidance with adult neurotics.

Before vocational guidance of any sort can be given, it is necessary to have what may be termed a vocational assessment. Immediately on admission, the chief psychiatrist assesses the patient's probable employability, a rating which we have seen correlates significantly with adjustment after discharge. The patient is then usually transferred to another doctor, who has charge of him throughout his stay in the Unit.

The patient is seen by the senior psychiatrist on the day of admission, and a full work record is taken. This is placed in the patient's case notes, and is available to other members of the staff, including the nurses, who have full access to the notes.

Shortly after this, the patient attends group psychological testing, where he receives Raven's Progressive Matrices (repeated individually where necessary), with no time limit. A day or two later he is given the Wechsler-Bellevue verbal scale as an individual test. These tests provide a rough estimate of the patient's functioning general intelligence. If there is any gross discrepancy in the results, further tests are given, as part of the routine testing procedure.

Later the psychologist has a number of interviews with each industrial patient, during which certain vocational and aptitude tests may be applied. Diagnostic psychological tests, such as the Rorschach and Thematic Apperception tests are given if requested by the patient's doctor.

In these interviews, employment difficulties and aspirations are discussed. On the basis of the test-results and the discussions the psychologist prepares his report on the apparent limits of the man's capacity, and suggests possible lines of approach in the search for suitable employment. The man's own wishes and interests play an important part in the psychologist's recommendations.

Soon after admission, one of the two Disablement Resettlement Officers of the Ministry of Labour (D.R.O.) sees the patient and discusses employment possibilities with him. The D.R.O. has at his interviews the patient's case notes, the work record assembled by the P.S.W., and the psychologist's report. Very often he has discussed the case informally with the other members of the staff who have dealings with the patient. The role of the D.R.O. has been presented elsewhere, and he fulfils a most important function. He is aware of the day-to-day fluctuations in the labour market, and of vacancies in Government training courses. He has up-to-date information on the number of jobs of any one type available in any particular area, and knows of specific work for which the patient could apply.

The D.R.O. uses the information he has from the other sources in directing his interview, but he also draws upon his own fund of experience in making suggestions to the patient. The D.R.O.'s report is written towards the end of the patient's stay in the Unit, and gives his opinion of the best placement possibilities.

Each patient is required to attend, for four hours daily one of the five workshops, unless he is excused attendance by his doctor. Freedom of choice of workshop is permitted, but the range of choice is limited by the number of vacant places in each shop. The workshops are not expressly designed as training centres, but (apart from their therapeutic function) provide an excellent means of assessing the patient in a work-situation. The instructor makes a weekly note of the patient's regularity of attendance, his relationship to the others in the shop, and the speed and quality of his work. A final and more comprehensive report is written shortly before the patient is due to be discharged.

A certain number of patients work in local firms for a period of about two hours each day. This provides an opportunity for a patient to practise a vocation in which he is interested, and thus to pave the way for full-time work. Similarly some patients are tried out in the Government training centre at Waddon, while still in the Unit.

One nurse has the full-time task of observing the patients at work in the shops, and of writing a report on each case before discharge. She also visits patients working for local firms, and keeps in close touch with their employers.

All the different reports are placed in the patient's case-notes, and it is the doctor who takes the decision that a patient should be discharged.

This decision is dependent firstly on the patient's psychiatric state, and secondly, on the availability of an apparently suitable job. A digest of each case is prepared by the psychiatrist, and sent to the patient's local employment exchange. This enables the officials there to have a clearer view of the difficulties and potentialities of the patient, should it be necessary for them to find him further jobs.

As a routine, patients are discussed at a weekly placement conference of the whole Unit staff. Here the doctor obtains advice and assistance in the placement of those cases which have proved difficult problems. The reports from each of the sources mentioned above are read out, and after discussion, a decision is usually reached. Every effort is made to place each patient directly from the Unit, and to minimize any delay between discharge and the start of work.

The problem of employability

If, as seems probable, patients vary along a scale of general adjustment which measures the extent to which they can cope with reality in the extra-hospital situation, then it seems equally probable that they can be ranged along a scale of potential adjustment, while still in hospital. This potential adjustment we have called 'employability', emphasizing the work-adjustment aspect because of its importance in relation to vocational assessment and guidance, and because of our concern in the Unit with this aspect of adjustment. In effect, an accurate assessment of a man's employability just before discharge from the Unit would predict his general adjustment after discharge. We may then define employability as the *capacity* for general adjustment.

The concept of employability was, we found, nothing new to the workshop instructors or the D.R.O.s. They had long been accustomed to distinguish between what they called 'good bets' and 'bad bets'. The 'good bet', with a high degree of employability, would be easily placed, and would have little difficulty in finding a suitable job—this, very often, without the aid of the psychologist or his tests. Such a patient could succeed in two quite dissimilar occupations, while the 'bad bet', on the other hand, is a constant headache to all concerned in his placement.

The psychologist and employability

The mean I.Q. of the Unit patients, derived from the Wechsler-Bellevue verbal scale, is 104, with a standard deviation of 16.6.

The frequency distribution for the Progressive Matrices is as follows:

	Cases
Grade I	26
Grade II	41
Grade III +	48
Grade III —	36
Grade IV	37
Grade V	24
Result unreliable or unobtainable	25
	237

The correlation of the Progressive Matrices score with adjustment, for ninety-two patients, is 0.188, which is statistically insignificant. The correlations of the Wechsler verbal section I.Q. and of the individual verbal sub-tests are even less, and it is quite clear that the intelligence tests used are not able to give us any estimate of employability; nor could the special aptitude tests, in the cases in which they were used.

Employability in the Unit population is a dimension which seems to be quite independent of intellectual factors, and which is without doubt a function of the patient's personality and psychiatric state.

What of the role of psychological tests in the case of the patient with a high employability? At first sight it would seem that, given the capacity for a good adjustment, psychological tests would help guide the patient into the most suitable vocation, to enable him to exploit his good employability in the most profitable way.

Experience with the Unit patients belies this completely. The 'good bet' who has improved during his stay, has no difficulty in finding a suitable job under conditions of full employment. His needs are met by discussion with his friends and family, and especially by the D.R.O.[1] who knows the exact state of the labour market in the man's home area. A high degree of employability enables the patient to find a suitable job, and what is more the *job he finds is interesting*. The 'bad bet' in spite of his abilities and aptitudes, finds no job suitable, and every job uninteresting. Patients may of course change during their stay in the Unit from 'bad' to 'good bets', which refers to their employability at any one time. Clearly it is the 'bad bet' who is constantly referred to the psychologist for guidance. Rather than face the fact that a patient has a low employability, those concerned in his placement turn with hope to the 'profile of abilities' offered by aptitude testing. Perhaps there exists some very special field in which this patient could make an adjustment. Perhaps he has some rare talent which would provide the solution to all his problems. It is probably these hopes that have perpetuated the use of aptitude tests with unemployed neurotics.

A further important fact has emerged in experience with unemployed neurotic patients. The interview and the test-situation are highly artificial, and it is extremely difficult in discussion to gauge the real level of employability. The patient may perform extremely well on all the tests, appear willing and keen to start work, and indeed may even have apparently reasonable ideas about what particular job he would like to do. The fact that he is a 'bad bet', as far as employability is concerned, may not be apparent to the investigator at all. It is probable that the psychologist's assessment is no more predictive than that of the psychiatrist (item 42). Suggested alternative methods of measuring employability will be discussed later in this chapter.

Vocational guidance without a knowledge of the patient's employability level, on the basis of tests and interview alone, may in fact be very much against the interests of the patient. For example, we had one case of an adolescent who had been advised, apparently on the basis of tests and interview, that he was fitted to be a courier, a steward, or a Customs' official. This advice was given while he was attending as an out-patient at a well-known psychiatric centre, and proved a serious difficulty in the way of finding him suitable employment. The patient's employability level was low, and yet he

---

[1] The D.R.O.'s value in this field cannot be over-estimated. The knowledge of the exact job-situation in the patient's home area is one of the most important bases for successful vocational guidance, and with this type of population, the conventional contribution of the psychologist is slight compared with that of the D.R.O.

fastened on these vocations as employment goals, for after all, did not the tests show that he was capable of being successful at any of the three occupations? His low employability was quite evident after a week or two as an in-patient, and he required a long term in hospital before his employability reached a level sufficiently high for him to be satisfactorily placed.

The nature of employability

There would appear to be a number of different factors which contribute to a low employability, and of these we may distinguish three which are specially important.

1. The diminution in working power caused by neurotic symptoms, e.g. compulsive actions, confusional symptoms, somatic complaints, etc.

2. Disturbance in social relations with employers and work mates, making it impossible to work with others.

3. Direct inhibition of work, in which the activity of work itself arouses such internal conflict, that, after a period of latency, inhibitions appear in relation to that work.

The fact that a latency period exists, is an extremely important one. Patients may appear to work well for a while, perhaps as long as a few weeks, before their work is affected by their low employability. This is one, perhaps, of the factors influencing the high labour turnover in certain occupations, and there must be a large body of workers who are compelled to change jobs within a given period of time, after work-inhibition has set in.

A number of cases in one of the Unit workshops were assessed daily[1] for several weeks, on a set of 11-point scales.[2] These scales were:

1. *Attitude to work:* Enthusiastic (+) vs. Apathetic (—).
2. *Social adjustment:* Gets on well (+) vs. Disliked (—).
3. *Aptitude for the work:* Picks it up easily (+) vs. Finds it difficult (—).

[1] The initiative for these assessments came from the bricklaying instructor, Mr. Strutton, who carefully and methodically assessed a number of patients daily for a period of some weeks.
[2] The signs (+) and (—) which follow, refer to the direction of high and low employability respectively, though these ratings were made before we had begun to think in terms of a scale of employability.

4. *Speed:* Very quick (+) vs. Very slow (—).
5. *Standard of work:* Very high (+) vs. Very poor (—).
6. *Persistence:* Does not give up easily (+) vs. Gives up easily (—).

The assessment of two cases is shown in Fig. 2.

Case 1 is aged twenty-five years, and was always very nervous. His difficulties were predominantly social and this affected his work. He was diagnosed as 'an inadequate personality with anxiety features'. This patient improved during his stay in the Unit, and greatly increased his capacity for mixing with others. The graphs showing his day-to-day change in the work situation indicate a constant improvement, and this was maintained for at least six months after discharge. At the follow-up visit he appeared happy and well settled in his new job.

Case 2, aged thirty-five years, had a history of never having held a job for long. He was a worrying and anxious type of person who lacked drive and persistence. He made no improvement in the hospital. In the bricklaying shop this patient constantly complained that the work was too difficult. On this account he was assigned a much simpler set of tasks, and an immediate improvement resulted. This lasted for less than three weeks, after which time he took up the same attitudes to his new tasks to those he had expressed in relation to the previous work. Six months after discharge this patient had shown no improvement and had tried several jobs with no success.

The measurement of employability

The correlations between certain items in the patient's work-record and general adjustment after discharge suggests that it is possible to estimate employability to some extent from each patient's history. These correlations are not high however, and a great deal of investigation is still needed to provide items which will give a better estimate of employability.

It is possible that certain questions could be found which would significantly relate to subsequent adjustment, and which could be taken together to give a fairly valid estimate of employability. These questions would refer either directly or indirectly, to the patient's attitude to work, and to his symptoms in the work-situation.

Most valuable of all would, I believe, be a model work-situation, in which the patient is observed for a period of not less than three weeks. In the bricklaying shop, for example, there are many grades and types of jobs possible, from simple labouring to complicated corner-work. It is not difficult to find a grade of job at which the patient works comfortably. If the man is of low general employ-

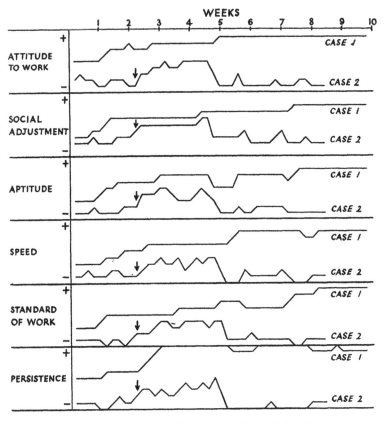

Fig. 2.—Graph showing change in adjustment in the workshop for two patients. The arrows indicate the point at which Case 2's work was changed (see text).

ability, the signs will soon appear. He will arrive late and depart early; he will stand around or chatter constantly with the others instead of attending to his work; he will find many excuses for absences during working hours, and the symptoms of which he complains will become increasingly severe. He may ask to be transferred to another shop, but inevitably the same cycle is repeated.[1] In many cases the patient works well for up to three weeks, and any assessment in the earlier part of his stay may be quite misleading.

The objection may be raised to these proposals, that patients may be uninterested in work that does not suit their particular pattern of abilities, and would work well at a suitable job. This objection, though it may be valid for other groups, does not, from our experience, hold with the neurotic unemployed.

---

[1] The workshop data reported earlier does not demonstrate these points clearly, although significant differences in the theoretically expected direction are found for item 46. The criteria of assessment were, at that time, ill-defined, due to our lack of experience and the fact that we were not at that time thinking in terms of employability.

CHAPTER X

GENERAL CONCLUSIONS

O ur findings appear to justify the conclusion that it is possible to change social attitudes in relatively desocialized patients with severe character disorders, provided they are treated together in a therapeutic community. Our results show that six months after leaving hospital two thirds of the patients followed up had made a fair adjustment or better, and one third were rated poor or very poor adjustments (Chapter VIII); just over one-half had worked the full time since leaving hospital. We believe (but cannot prove) that the results described could not have been achieved by individual psychotherapy and hospitalization alone.

From the follow-up results there would appear to be a tendency for the patients to make either good or bad adjustments. This tendency is demonstrated by the shape of the distribution of adjustment scores shown in Fig. 1, Chapter VIII.

It would appear that our patient population is composed of two main types, those who derive much benefit from treatment and those who improve but little; there are relatively few patients who fall between these two groups (only 18 per cent of our patients have adjustment scores in the range 2 to 7).

Those patients who showed clinical improvement in hospital, irrespective of the severity of their illness on admission, do significantly better as a group than those who show no comparable improvement in hospital. Thus a very ill patient who improves considerably in hospital has a tendency to a better prognosis than a mildly ill patient who shows relatively slight improvement. This may imply much more than symptomatic improvement. It usually went with change in social adjustment, attitude to work, etc. It is worth stressing that it is the capacity of the individual for change, rather than the severity of his illness, which is the important factor in estimating prognosis. This may possibly modify current concepts regarding the assessment in the initial interviews of the outcome of treatment.

Dr. Sandler's work on vocational guidance with our type of patient suggests that too much emphasis has in the past been placed on the patient's abilities and aptitudes as measured by psychological tests. Attention should rather be directed to an assessment of the patient's 'general employability' (see Chapter IX) which determines the patient's attitude to work as such. A high general employability implies that the patient will have little difficulty in adjusting to whatever work is available to him. Conversely a person with a low general employability will not succeed in keeping a job no matter how favourable the initial prospects may have seemed.

There are many people who doubt the value of in-patient treatment of the neuroses; what appears to us to be important is the organization of the hospital community. Clearly every general hospital, mental hospital, or neurosis centre has some form of social structure, but all too frequently this has been established on intuitive, empirical or dictatorial grounds. Too little attention has been paid to the effect of the hospital community on the individual patient. Even less has any serious attempt been made to use the hospital community as an active force in treatment. (The Cassel Hospital near London is one exception to this.) We have tried to build up a therapeutic community where each member of the staff has a clear concept of his or her role. By frequent (daily) meetings of the staff, these roles have been elaborated and clarified and the inter-personal relationships developed by discussion and by resolution of tensions where possible. The social structure of the Unit has become a relatively integrated one and has stood firm in the face of serious threats to its existence from both inside and outside the Unit. The traditions and culture of the staff group have become more sharply defined in relation to the treatment needs of the patients. The Unit culture is more clearly seen and understood in the staff group, but the majority of patients are influenced by it to a considerable extent. The patients come to us as social casualties; they are mainly people who have no real place in society coming as they do from broken homes and being unemployed. We attempt to absorb them into a hospital group where everything is done to find them social and vocational roles. As far as possible the workshops simulate normal factory conditions where the tensions associated with work roles can be worked out while still in hospital. In this sense the Unit is a transitional community. The nurses play an important role being accepted by both staff and patient groups—more than any other members of the staff they can be said to transmit the culture of the Unit to the patients.

A nurse trained in general nursing or in a mental hospital has in addition to her various skills come to accept certain traditions regarding say the nurse-patient relationship, the nurse-doctor relationship, and so on. It is probable that most of these traditions have never been subjected to close scrutiny; hospitals in Britain have in general remained peculiarly ignorant of developments in the sociological field. On the Unit we have tried to be as objective as possible in developing our therapeutic community and to become conscious of our motives when establishing a pattern of behaviour expected from the staff or patients. Along with this we have paid special attention to communications throughout the entire Unit population, together with free discussion of any problem affecting the community. This has meant a considerable distribution of responsibility, e.g. at a staff meeting a nurse may describe one of her disturbed patients whom she considers to be unsuitable for nursing in an open ward. Her previous training in a general or mental hospital has led her to expect that the doctor will 'do something', which in this case would probably mean removing the patient to a closed ward (usually a mental hospital). In the staff meeting the nurse finds herself playing an entirely different role. She is expected to consider the problem as one which if possible, we should resolve within the Unit; certainly the doctor is not prepared to solve it for her on his own. He wants to know what, in her opinion, has contributed to the exacerbation of symptoms (if that has occurred), while he on his side will discuss any factors which in his opinion have contributed to the disturbed state of the patient. Other nurses who have been looking after the patient may express divergent views and the meeting may become aware that considerable tension exists between the several nurses handling the patient. The workshop instructor may tell the group that the patient has become increasingly more hostile towards the other patients, and along with this has sought more and more attention and praise from the instructor. The charge nurse too may have noticed that he has been in her office more often than previously, and frequently with quite trivial requests. The social worker may describe the patient's appalling home conditions and the complete indifference of his parents to his condition—no help can be expected from this direction. At this point the nurse who originally raised the problem may feel that the tension is unbearable and may interject angrily, 'Why don't you *do* something about it instead of all this talking? In my last hospital Dr. Smith would have acted immediately.' Such action if taken would not necessarily resolve the nurse's anxiety. There might be an immediate feeling of relief for the nurse but all too frequently the guilt engendered by such actions appears later in critical remarks by the nurse about the doctor, who is accused of showing no real interest in his patients and so on. Our aim is to achieve a communal responsibility in relation to all our Unit problems whether they relate to patients or staff. This distribution of responsibility while frequently increasing the tensions, particularly of the less trained and more dependent members of the staff, leads to a far more realistic attitude towards treatment.

We have come to feel that it is high time that hospital communities throughout the country became more conscious of their treatment roles. All too often established practice bears no relationship to the treatment needs of the patient. In many instances they appear to be an elaborate defence protecting the staff against such needs. Take any acute surgical ward with say, several recent amputees; the staff are gay and inconsequential and expect an appropriate response from the patients. It is not until the patients have returned home that they can talk about the very real problems that now face them. The staff have protected themselves from facing responsibilities that they shrink from, and moreover this is part of the established tradition of 'good nursing'; but one of the major aspects of treatment, the patients own emotional problems, has been ignored. We believe that the application of some of the principles of sociology such as we have described, would favourably alter the existing social structure of hospital communities with considerable benefit to the patient.

In many psychiatric hospitals which I have visited in the U.S.A. and Europe while acting as Consultant in Mental Health to the World Health Organization, I have seen what appears to be a most sincere attempt to give the patient the best possible treatment, spoilt by a failure to distinguish between a hospital role and a normal community role. In these hospitals everything possible was done to make the patient's stay pleasant and interesting; even when the patient was nearing discharge, the planned day was designed to please him rather than to prepare him for his outside role. The result of this was that frequently the patient was unable to settle down when discharged to his home, and he soon found his way back to the hospital. On the Unit we have tried to avoid this error and have stressed the ultimate job goal from the time of the patient's admission. The cultural pressure of the Unit community is directed towards his acceptance of a more useful social role, which may then appear desirable because of his growing identification with the group. This insistence on a work goal is much more unpleasant for both patients and staff than the more usual type of hospital environment but it is more realistic, and probably yields better results in the long run.

We believe that too little use is made of educational methods in psychiatric hospitals. Our use of daily discussion groups with the entire patient population, documentary films, psychodramas, etc., represent an attempt to develop such methods; the main principle involved is that social problems and real life situations are either raised in discussion or acted out in psychodrama. The whole group attempts to arrive at a constructive attitude in relation to the problem raised. The degree of participation by the doctor taking the meeting varies with the situation and the personality of the doctor, but in his summing up he has an opportunity to present an informed and comprehensive point of view. To take the patient population repeatedly through this type of discussion or acting out of real life situations does possibly give them a new perception of such situations and so may alter behaviour patterns; this new awareness may prove helpful in dealing with the patient's own problems. The awareness may not amount to actual insight, but the very process of acting out or verbalization of feelings and attitudes gives definition to them, and in so doing modifies them. However, in our educational procedure individual responses cannot be separated from the group climate. What appears to matter most is the degree of 'group learning'—the extent to which the community accepts an idea which then becomes an integral part of the group culture. Patients seem to accept new ideas much more readily when these have behind them the weight of group acceptance. This attempt to achieve a change in the attitude of a group was discussed in Chapter I in relation to cardiac neurosis. Cases of effort syndrome (neurocirculatory asthenia) were treated in a group and fed with information of an anatomical and physiological kind, sufficient to give them a mechanistic understanding of the nature of their symptoms. The group ingested the information and in time the attitude of the group changed significantly. Originally every man had thought of his symptoms as a demonstration of severe heart disease; but this attitude slowly changed and was replaced by a more mechanistic view which disallowed the possibility of heart disease. The symptoms might persist but their significance was now completely altered. New patients rapidly came to accept this orientation which had become part of the culture of the group, and was discussed by the patients at the daily community meetings, and in this way was perpetuated. This process of acculturation seems to be an essential part of our social therapy techniques. We realize only too well the limitations of such treatment procedures. There are probably some patients who remain unaffected by the group meetings. Moreover there must be other patients who are unlikely to be helped by anything but uncovering types of psychotherapy. It must be borne in mind, however, that we are dealing with severe character disorders with poor personalities, who would in most cases be quite unsuitable for analytic types of treatment.

At the present time we believe it is necessary to get the severe character disorder of the type discussed in this book, into a therapeutic community in order to effect some degree of resocialization; however, we have been impressed by Miss Tuxford's experiences in doing the home visits for the follow-up study; these led her to the conclusion that the cause of much of the desocialization which we see in hospital is due to the absence of any real family life. It may be that we would be able to do more useful work if we were keeping the patient at home and attempting treatment within the home environment as is being done by the psychiatrists and social workers in the Amsterdam Municipal Health Service and in other Dutch cities. Moreover we have so far failed to bring the patients' families into our community treatment, mainly because we get patients from all over the United Kingdom. We believe that our experiment might yield more valuable information if we were serving only the local community. Whatever the advantages of working within the family environment may be, however, we feel certain that there is ample therapeutic justification for bringing patients into a therapeutic community until other and better methods of treatment are known. There is no reason to think that the changes in social attitude which the patient follow-up inquiry demonstrated, and the striking differences in this sphere between the treated and untreated groups, were temporary phenomena. Admittedly the follow-up done six months after the patient having left hospital is too short a period of time on which to base any final conclusions; the social worker's impression, however, was that the greater social awareness of the treated group would persist. We would very much like to do a second follow-up after a period of say two years to test this point.

Our attempts to have matched treated and untreated groups for the follow-up inquiry failed despite the utmost co-operation from the Ministry of Labour. In any sociological studies the difficulties of obtaining scientifically valid control groups are almost insuperable. Nevertheless the follow-up study of the untreated group was well worth while and provided a useful background against which to evaluate the changes in social attitudes in the treated group. It also helped to draw attention to an important sociological group which needs further study: the type of unemployed neurotic who would not consider going into hospital for treatment. We have always been aware of the existence of such casualties and although we have aimed at admitting the most 'hopeless' chronic neurotic unemployed person to the Unit, we have known that even our population was in a sense a selected one; we were not getting the patient who refused to be helped and would never go to a doctor at all. It may be that such patients could be helped by the Family Service Units which in Britain are attempting to penetrate into even the worst homes of squalor and apathy and reconstitute such families. The number of psychotic patients 'discovered' in this disabled person follow-up, who were not receiving any form of treatment or supervision, emphasized the need for better social after-care services in Britain.

Finally this study of a sample of registered disabled unemployed persons highlighted the difficulties facing the Ministry of Labour Disablement Resettlement Officer in Britain. The D.R.O. is frequently called upon to help in the resettlement of those extremely difficult problems. He may have no one to turn to for help except perhaps an overworked general practitioner. In Britain an attempt is being made to set up Medical Interviewing Committees in all the large towns where problem cases can be referred by the D.R.O. for an expert medical opinion, but there are still too few such committees, largely due to the lack of co-operation from the medical profession. We believe, however, that even such provision would be inadequate in the type of case under discussion. With difficult psychological problems a period of observation in a hospital environment is often necessary before deciding on the man's disability and rehabilitation prospects. Government officials and others sometimes desire, for reasons of expediency, to label individuals as 'unemployable'; in our opinion this is frequently impossible unless the individual has been observed under hospital conditions for weeks if not months. However, the fact remains that complex cases of this character are frequently dealt with by the D.R.O. alone, because he has no expert help available. The D.R.O. cannot be expected to deal with anything beyond the man's employment problems, and in difficult cases he must have help available from all the skills in the rehabilitation field. The establishment of Industrial Resettlement Units in the twelve big towns in Britain has gone a long way to supplying this need, but as our follow-up shows, much still remains to be done. Our own experience, working alongside two D.R.O.s, seconded to us full time by the Ministry of Labour, has been that they are as important in a rehabilitation team, as are the psychiatrists themselves.

In conclusion we feel that this study has demonstrated the possibilities of treatment with patients who were generally regarded as being both untreatable and unemployable. We hope that we have contributed in some small way to the social psychiatric treatment of such cases.

ADDENDUM

IN the following account we have attempted to illustrate how patients' social attitudes may be changed by the use of community methods of treatment.

The sum of £30 was stolen from the social worker's office on 11th February, 1952. During the next five weeks several minor thefts of clocks, etc., occurred in the wards, and on 17th March a patient announced that £5 had been stolen from his suitcase. These events created considerable anxiety in the patient population who adopted a rather passive attitude and clearly felt that it was the responsibility of the staff to relieve their anxiety. We, however, felt that it was a problem affecting the whole community and during the next ten days we used this topic as the central theme for our community meetings. We believe that considerable change occurred in the community's attitude towards antisocial behaviour such as theft, and also in their attitude to 'informing'.

Several volunteer members of the staff acted as reporters and made notes during and after the proceedings. The secretary made a verbatim shorthand record of the 9 a.m. meetings. During the ten days covered by this record the meetings conformed to the usual pattern of the Unit programme as described in Chapters 2, 3 and 4. There was a daily meeting of all patients and staff from 9 a.m. to 9.45 a.m., in which group projection techniques and discussion methods were used. In addition, two-thirds of the patient population were in therapeutic groups of eight to ten patients which met from two to four times a week and discussions developed at the 9 a.m. meeting tended to be continued in these groups. There were also administrative ward meetings for each of the three wards in the Unit and these were sometimes held at 8.30 a.m. so that a topic developed in the ward could be further discussed with the whole community at 9 a.m. The staff met, without the patients, every day at 9.45 a.m. to discuss and evaluate the reactions occurring in the patient population in the preceding meeting. The staff also met three times a week for one hour to plan the 9 a.m. meetings and clarify the staff attitude to the various social problems raised by the patients. This meeting and the nurses' tutorials with the doctors afforded an opportunity for the pooling of information regarding the reaction of individual patients to the current problems. Information from all these sources is included in the following account. We cannot claim to have an accurate assessment of the social changes which occurred in the patients individually or in the community as a whole. To attempt this we clearly need the services of an experienced social anthropologist. Nevertheless, this account represents the considered opinion of thirty staff members, who by virtue of the structure of the Unit, have a considerable degree of social penetration into the patient population.

Monday 17th March, 9.0 a.m. Meeting
This meeting opened as usual with an account by the chairman of the Patients' Entertainments Committee of the current week's social activities, and a statement of the club's finances. When he came to the latter, Mr. A. explained with considerable emotion that the funds had been stolen from his suitcase. He held up the battered case which was made of some cheap composition material and had been ripped open. There was a gasp of amazement from the audience and in response to Mr. A.'s emotion came an immediate chorus of reassuring voices all telling him that he was in no way to blame. Mr. A. went on to say that he knew he should have deposited the money in the Sister's office, that in his past life he had handled large sums of money, but this was the first time he had ever been responsible for any loss. The group, having apparently exonerated Mr. A., now looked round for a scapegoat. Some patients wanted to call the police, others implied that the staff were to blame as they never did anything to protect the community, and the growing list of thefts over the past five weeks demonstrated clearly how they had failed to meet the problem. Other patients reminded the community that on a recent occasion when a patient had insisted on the police being called in, the result had been completely negative. One psychiatrist suggested that we follow the pattern adopted since the time of the £30 theft, and that we must regard the theft as a symptom of an illness and focus our attention on treatment rather than on punishment. Another enlarged on this and asked the patients to cooperate by passing on any relevant information to the staff, just as they would in the case of any other illness such as epilepsy. The

social worker used this opportunity to stress that the community could often help the individual by informing her about other patients' economic or social distress, because often the patients themselves might hold back information. Such distress might even be a contributory factor in an impulse to steal. Everyone seemed to feel that the time available was too short to allow a full discussion and it was agreed to continue the meeting at 9 a.m. on Tuesday.

At the 9.45 a.m. meeting of the staff, we agreed that, although our staff attitude towards theft might be a legitimate one and might even be shared by a part of the patient population, it had clearly failed to get the whole community to accept it as *their* problem. We thought that the 9 a.m. meeting had shown that the patients' attitude towards an 'informer' was in line with a schoolboy's attitude to 'telling tales' and they still acted as though to inform was to invoke a punitive rather than a therapeutic situation. We decided that for the remainder of the week we would try to increase the community's awareness of its responsibility as the only way to deal with the present state of uncertainty and fear. Essentially, we had to try to alter the patient community's attitude to informing and improve our communications. We agreed to attempt a further evaluation of the patients' attitudes towards informing and also to attempt to assess their reaction to the staff's cultural attitude to stealing. We felt that one way to do this was to ask specific questions in the therapeutic groups of eight to ten patients if the problems were not raised spontaneously.

In one group, all the patients expressed the opinion that in the present situation the proper procedure was to convey any relevant information to the staff, but there was a clearly expressed anxiety that such communications must be treated as confidential otherwise reprisals of an unpleasant nature might ensue. However, further discussion seemed to convince the group that the community's strength and goodwill would be sufficient to protect them no matter what happened. Approval was expressed of the staff's cultural attitude towards theft, but it was felt that when the individual or individuals were known, they would have to co-operate much more fully in treatment than they appeared to have done to date. The group implied that the individual's refusal to seek his doctor's help regarding his impulse to steal was an index of his unwillingness to be helped. If this attitude were to persist, then the group indicated that the patient or patients should be discharged from hospital.

Another group also appeared to feel that any relevant information about antisocial behaviour ought to be made available to the staff, but one patient felt that she would first communicate her intention to the individual concerned. There was not the same general agreement regarding the staff's cultural attitude towards theft. Three patients felt that it was sensible and that they had come to accept this outlook, but three other patients felt that it was too idealistic, and some form of punishment was needed. Another patient felt that it was entirely a matter for the police and had nothing to do with either the staff or patients. Mr. A. was a member of this group and was accused by another patient of dramatizing his loss. This led to a split in the group, some being for and others against Mr. A. This patient professed to identify himself entirely with the staff's attitude towards theft, and was the only patient in the two groups who claimed to have held this attitude even before admission to hospital.

In another group all the patients but one spoke in favour of full communication with the staff in the event of antisocial behaviour by another patient.

Tuesday 18th March, 9.0 a.m. Meeting

Yesterday's discussion, regarding the loss of the club funds and the other recent thefts, was continued at the 9 a.m. meeting. The staff were again attacked and it was suggested that they were to blame as they had not taken the necessary extra precautions following the initial theft five weeks previously. The Unit's secretary suggested that she was partly to blame as she had not taken full responsibility for the club's money; this had been decided at the staff meeting following the £30 theft, but the secretary had been ill since that time and had made an appointment to see Mr. A. and collect the club money on Monday 17th March. A patient said that this still showed the careless attitude adopted by the staff, and the staff accepted this criticism as just. Another patient said that he had changed his mind since yesterday and now felt that people should communicate anything they knew or suspected regarding thefts to the staff. This attitude was opposed by other patients. One patient felt that the whole discussion was pointless, and that the problem had nothing to do with illness; the culprit should be found by the police and it was for them to decide whether he needed punishment or treatment. A psychiatrist pointed out that unless the patients were willing to help the police they were relatively impotent as were the staff; in fact we were unlikely to achieve very much until such time as the community adopted the problem as its own.

At the 9.45 a.m. meeting of the staff, it was agreed that there had been active interest among the patients but relatively little participation. One member felt that a sociodramatic technique such as we usually have on a Tuesday would have resulted in more overt feeling and participation. Another felt that as we know so little about learning processes, it was premature to assume that a projection technique which aroused considerable feeling was more likely to effect a change in attitude than a more factual appeal to reason. The psychologist remarked that although some thirty patients in therapeutic groups had spoken yesterday of the need to the staff, practically no one had openly supported this view in the 9 a.m. meeting to-day.

In a therapeutic group of seven patients, two felt that informing on other patients was justified if it helped the patients; two felt that it would depend on whether they were friends or not; another would definitely inform; another would 'have it out privately with the offender'; and the last member said he had been day dreaming and did not know what it was all about.

Wednesday 19th March, 9.0 a.m. Meeting

It was decided to use a projection technique to bring out the problem of poor communication between patients and staff. An out-patient psychiatric clinic was chosen as the setting and the doctor's role was played by one of the psychiatrists, the nurses filling three other roles. One was the nurse on duty at the clinic, another the patient, and a third the patient's mother. The final role of probation officer was played by the Unit secretary. The patient was a delinquent girl, aged nineteen, who had been found by the police in a stolen car driven by her brother. The brother had been sent to prison for three months and the girl had been put on probation for a year on condition that she received psychiatric treatment. When ushered into the doctor's office by the nurse, the girl on probation proved to be a cheeky adolescent, contemptuous of psychiatry, and in no way interested in treatment. She frequently refused to answer questions and was thoroughly unco-operative. The psychiatrist explained that he was not concerned with punishment but wanted only to help her. This made no impression on the girl who had said that she wasn't sick, so why did she need treatment? She refused to consider the possibility of coming into hospital. At this point she was asked to wait in the waiting-room and nurse brought in her mother. The latter was even more guarded and uncommunicative than her daughter. She didn't believe in this 'psychology stuff' and there was nothing wrong with her daughter. She refused to divulge any facts relating to her daughter's past or present mode of life, nor would she talk about her son now in prison.

The probation officer was interviewed next. She said that the family lived in a very bad district which had recently been terrorised by a gang of adolescents who had committed many robberies with violence, etc. Conditions were such that the police patrolled the district in pairs. There was no father, the mother drank, and the two children seemed to do pretty well what they liked. However, the probation officer could not furnish much information as she too was met by a solid resistance by both mother and daughter.

At this point the psychiatrist turned to the audience and asked them to think of themselves as doctors faced with this problem and invited them to carry on with the conduct of the case.

Mr. J., a patient, who was himself on probation, said that he'd been interviewed by a psychiatrist under similar circumstances and the doctor here had not been paternal enough; so he was asked to come forward and assume the psychiatrist's role. This he did quite cheerfully and faced by the delinquent girl he proceeded to try to make friends with her. He explained the difficult position in which he as a doctor was placed when a patient refused to co-operate. He only wanted to help and understand her; but he failed to get any response. He then asked to see the girl's mother, but again was met by a negativistic attitude. Nor could the probation officer offer him much help; she was finding it almost impossible to get any rapport with either mother or daughter. The daughter was called back and the 'doctor' pleaded with her to go into hospital, but the delinquent simply walked out of the office ignoring his protests.

The psychiatrist summed up by pointing out that we had just seen how helpless both psychiatry and the law were in face of unco-operative and uncommunicative behaviour on the part of the patient and her mother. If the treatment situation failed to develop because of this negativistic attitude then the probation officer might be forced to report the girl to the magistrate, who might well punish her. The situation had much in common with our current Unit problem.

At the 9.45 a.m. meeting of the staff it was felt that despite the absence of comment many of the patients might have realized that we were bringing out our current problem and underlining the staff's impotence if the patients would not accept their responsibility too. The wisdom of the psychiatrist's summing-up was questioned and the Sister (charge nurse) felt that this simply produced a negativistic attitude in the patients. The psychiatrist himself felt that while the projection technique certainly aroused interest and feeling it needed a summing up to conceptualize it. In other words that if learning did occur it might be thought that the feeling and intellectual processes were complementary.

One group discussed the 9 a.m. meeting quite spontaneously. Half the group said that they had realized that the theme was the current Unit problem even before the psychiatrist's summing up. One patient expressed anxiety about the community's attitude towards the culprit if he were actually found. People might say now that he needed treatment not punishment, but if the vague concept of 'someone' were to become a particular person the climate of opinion might suddenly harden. Even if the whole situation were dealt with as confidential, the secret would almost inevitably leak out.

In another group the topic of the 9 a.m. meeting was also raised spontaneously and most of the patients felt that the relationship to the Unit's current problem was obvious. They still maintained that it was desirable for staff-patient communication to be as free as possible.

Another group participated freely, much more so than on any previous occasion, every member speaking and sometimes quite heatedly. The eight members of the group all said that they would inform a doctor if they had relevant information, but it was clear that not all of them had really accepted the staff concept. One stressed that he did not want the police to be called in because of his own previous record and would prefer that the Senior Psychiatrist be given all information so that he might act as the 'policeman' of the Unit. One patient expressed the view that he would not feel responsible if, having withheld information, further thefts occurred, and another patient said he would feel very guilty if information given by him made things worse.

A fourth group had its first meeting of the week. They were asked to comment on their feeling regarding the staff attitude towards informing and also the change, if any, in their own attitude toward the problem of theft. There was no decisive feeling in answer to the first question. One patient said he felt the staff was too lenient. Four felt that treating the £30 loss as a symptom has encouraged thieving. One patient wanted to blame someone outside the Unit, a 'visitor'. There was a general agreement that it is hard to reconcile past experiences of punishment with the staff attitude. All but one patient expressed a wish that the staff should deal with this type of problem without involving the patients. One patient said he thought the staff attitude was the correct one and he had come to believe in it since coming to hospital. Another patient said he would not contribute to any ward collection until the Unit's money problem had been straightened out. They all said they would give information if they had it. They also brought out that as they all slept in either Ward A or Ward C, they felt that Ward B was under suspicion. However, since the thefts they had become more distrustful of each other in their own wards.

At the 1 p.m. staff meeting it was agreed that if the patients raised the question of making good the £5 loss, we would oppose it. It was felt that in making good the £30 loss, we had given some of the patients the impression that their financial problems would be settled by the staff, so there was no need for the patients to worry. It might even act as an invitation for further stealing. The patients' financial interests must, however, be safeguarded and from now on we would act as their bankers, and any loss would be our responsibility.

Thursday, 20th March, 9 a.m. Meeting

For this meeting it was decided again to use a projection technique. It was felt that the difficulty in confessing should be highlighted as otherwise we could only treat the individual concerned indirectly as an unknown member of the community.

A family scene was enacted with the psychiatrist as the son, the Unit Sister as the mother, and two nurses as the sisters. The mother suggested that as it was a holiday they should go for a picnic, but the son would have to be left behind as he was not well enough for such an outing. The son did not object and the mother praised him excessively and stressed how he was always such a good boy. When the others had gone the son sat reading for a while and then, on looking up, noticed his mother's purse and helped himself to half-a-crown. Then the family returned tired but pleased after a successful trip. The mother needed some money, took her purse and noticed with surprise that half-a-crown was missing. She asked the girls if they knew anything about it but they did not; however, they told the mother that their brother had remarked recently that he needed some money. The son immediately denied having opened his mother's purse. The psychiatrist now turned to the audience and asked for comments. It was suggested that the son was resentful because the family left him alone; also that the sisters were trying to exclude him from the family group and would be glad to incriminate him in the theft, etc. Eventually, Mr. M. suggested that the son (played by the psychiatrist) should confess. He went to the family to confess, but in fact he did not. This provoked consideration of the difficulty in any confession and the audience seemed to warm up. Someone suggested that the mother was a difficult person who by forcing a 'good' role on her son made it difficult for him to confess. Some patients felt that it would be best to confess, but others disagreed. Mr. M. suggested that the son should put the money back without anybody knowing. This was then acted out and it was demonstrated that the sisters' suspicion persisted and the family still quarrelled. The audience again discussed why it was difficult to confess. The son was advised to try and make the mother's attitude towards him more realistic. This was acted out, the son telling her that he was not so good as she thought, and pointing out that her attitude made everyone expect too much of him and also annoyed his sisters. The son then appeared to be on the verge of confessing when he broke off and turned to the audience. The latter was by now participating freely at a feeling level and urged the son to confess: this seemed to be clearly the feeling of the community as a whole. The son now returned to the family and confessed; and the family's reactions were demonstrated and discussed. Some patients pointed out that until the thief confessed suspicion would tend to fall on the innocent. These patients came from the ward which was associated with the recent thefts. The psychiatrist (who had played the role of the son) now summed up and pointed out that the thief in our midst had been asked to play the difficult role of confessor; nevertheless it seemed to be the only constructive thing for him to do and the only way in which the 'family' tension could be eased. He pointed out that the confession had been made more difficult because the son had been looked on as the 'good boy'. Mr.

M. pointed out the difficulty of confession for those who were 'bad boys' and were expected to do wrong.

At the 9.45 a.m. meeting of the staff everyone felt that the audience had wanted the thief to confess, but it was also clear that a public confession of this kind would be extremely difficult for the person concerned; also that secrecy would be difficult to obtain or maintain. The psychiatrist felt that he had achieved his objective in obtaining the patients' participation and their expressed need to have a confession in order to relieve the family tension. At this point he thought it might be better on future occasions to let a patient, or several patients, playing the part of the son, do the confessing. Such acting out might have established a pattern of behaviour and made it easier for the real thief to confess. Moreover, he thought that the family should have received the confession with relief and brought out some underlying motives for the theft so that the idea of understanding and 'treatment' rather than punishment was stressed. This had not been done because the family scene had only been roughly sketched with the staff before the 9 a.m. meeting and there had been no actual rehearsal or elaboration of a definite goal.

One therapeutic group discussed the 9 a.m. meeting spontaneously. They felt sorry for the boy who was left behind when the family went to the seaside. The whole group tended to reproach the family for the son's theft. One patient felt that the son had stolen in order to get more attention from his family. Nurse asked if the same explanation might apply to the individual who had stolen the Unit's funds. This was discussed at length and it was felt that the culprit might feel that the community here was too permissive and nice, and had wanted to disturb it or to attract attention to himself.

Another group also raised the topic of the 9 a.m. meeting spontaneously, and said that they had developed a good understanding of the reasons for confession but found it difficult to picture themselves actually doing this if they were personally involved.

Two groups declined to discuss the 9 a.m. meeting.

Friday 21st March. Psychodrama
This is performed every Friday by a volunteer patient who starts rehearsing with his own chosen cast a week beforehand. Under the circumstances it is not usually part of a planned theme for the week and for that reason is not discussed here.

Monday 24th March, 9 a.m. Meeting

The chairman of the Patients' Entertainments Committee opened the proceedings as usual, but had nothing of particular interest to report. The psychiatrist then asked for any suggestions or criticisms which might help to direct us in the organization and running of the Unit. The main topic was misuse of the expensive radiogram used for the patients' socials, etc. It was agreed that in future this should be kept locked and the responsibility for its proper use be left in the hands of the Patients' Entertainments Committee. One of the patients who in the meetings of the previous week had identified himself with the staff's attitude toward current problems, apologized to the group for getting drunk and coming in late over the week-end. The psychiatrist thanked him, but the patients made no comment.

9.45 a.m. Meeting

The Unit Sister felt that the patients were in a restless and ambivalent emotional state. A nurse remarked on the absence of free participation in the discussion at the 9 a.m. meeting. There was, we felt, a general feeling of tension.

In one group a member suggested that the average patient said nothing at the 9 a.m. meeting because he was afraid of upsetting other patients' feelings or of making enemies. The question was raised whether patients were justified in remaining silent; if they accepted the staff ideology would it not be more desirable to say so and not allow the more antisocial patients to appear to be more representative of the community than they actually were? There seemed to be general agreement on this point.

In another group the question of the 'silent' members of the 9 a.m. meetings was raised again. Three patients spoke quite vehemently about their fear of reprisals if they complained about the antisocial behaviour of patients. They talked about a 'certain patient' in Ward B who had been responsible for at least two acts of violence on little or no pretext. They went on to discuss Ward B and Mr. C. said that it was split into two parts, one half making tea, etc., and dominating the ward kitchen, while the other half was made to understand that it was unwanted in such activities. Other patients agreed with this point of view. Nurse then asked why they did not complain and was told that they feared reprisals.

At the 1 p.m. staff meeting it was agreed that the topic for the week should be the place of public opinion in countering a minority 'gangster' rule in the community. It was decided that the psychiatrist should see Ward B at 8.30 a.m. the following morning in the hope that they would discuss the 'split' and that an attempt should be made to continue this meeting at the 9 a.m. meeting of the whole Unit community. On further discussion it appeared that two of the nurses had been afraid to report on Mr. M. This patient had been discussed many times at staff meetings and the suggestion had been made several times during the previous four months that as he was such a disrupting influence on the community, he should be discharged. However, in the end it had always been agreed that we should persevere with treatment as rejection by us would in all probability result in the patient turning to a life of crime. It now appeared that Mr. M. had frightened the nurses by 'playfully' pulling their cloak ends round their necks until they felt faint. The social worker pointed out that the nurses were doing just what the patients appeared to be doing and by not communicating such anti-social behaviour they were probably encouraging the more aggressive patient element to further excesses. The psychiatrist added that such physical contact witnessed by other patients probably affected the attitude of patients to nurses to a greater degree than was commonly appreciated. After prolonged discussion it was decided that as Mr. M. was not apparently benefiting from treatment, was certainly not co-operating with the staff, and was disrupting the community life, he should be asked to leave hospital. This procedure was agreed to by his psychiatrist and Mr. M. was interviewed and provided with the necessary travel warrant to return home the next day. It was explained to him that he was not being discharged as a punishment but simply because we felt that we had done all we could to help him. He appeared to accept his discharge with a good grace.

That night three men were seen on the hospital roof about 11 p.m., but escaped when challenged. The police were informed immediately and arrived within a few minutes, but there was no sign of any intruders, and all the patients appeared to be accounted for in the wards.

Tuesday 25th March, 8.30 a.m. Meeting

Ward B was usually seen by a psychiatrist on Fridays and was asked to meet on the Tuesday because he had been unable to meet them at all the previous week. Nevertheless they were overtly hostile and suspicious and insisted that they had no problems to discuss. (Mr. M. who was leaving that day did not attend the meeting.) The psychiatrist said that the nurses on the ward reported that there was some disagreement among the patients regarding the distribution of tea, but the patients denied any such trouble or division of the ward into two camps. Their resentment was then directed towards the staff, both doctors and the nurses; ward meetings were a waste of time as nothing was ever done about their complaints and so on. At the last meeting ten days previously they had complained about the lavatory windows, but nothing had been done to rectify their complaint, etc. Despite the hostile atmosphere, the ward with but two exceptions agreed to co-operate in the 9 a.m. meeting. (The patients, who had described the tension in their ward in a group meeting the previous day, remained silent during this ward meeting.)

9 a.m. Meeting

The Unit community was told that Ward B had kindly agreed to continue their discussion as though they were still alone in their ward. Mr. C. started a long dissertation about the tea group in Ward B who monopolized the ward kitchen and cornered all the milk. He compared Ward B unfavourably with Ward A where everyone appeared to be happy and there was a family atmosphere. Ward A interrupted periodically and exposed the split in Ward B with obvious enjoyment. Eventually someone in Ward B said that Mr. C. would never have been allowed to talk like that in the real ward meeting and that Mr. C. was addressing the Unit as a whole and not Ward B only. Mr. L. then pointed out that, whereas at 8.30 a.m. meeting they had said there was no ward problem, now it was clear that there *was* a problem and he added his own version of the split. Several other 'silent members' of Ward B now became articulate and met with considerable hostility from the dominant element in the ward. The leader of this dominant set was always referred to anonymously. (He was well known to the staff, and was closely associated with Mr. M., who was leaving that day, as one of the aggressive leaders of the ward.) The dominant element in the ward said that they had no wish to monopolize the tea and the others were welcome to use the kitchen, etc., but they must provide their own tea (which is strictly rationed in the U.K.). There was much hostility expressed towards the staff and the psychiatrist in particular by Ward B. They repeated that when the ward meeting was announced they immediately felt that there was some crisis as the meetings were never held on that day. The psychiatrist summed up by drawing attention to the fear of reprisals which led to many ward members remaining silent despite the existence of real problems; this state of affairs was linked with the current Unit problem of thefts and the question of social responsibility compared with a false sense of loyalty or fear of reprisals in a community which was afraid of its dominant elements.

9.45 a.m. Meeting

Everyone agreed that the patients had had a good demonstration of the importance of free communication if group tensions were to be resolved. The psychiatrist reported that after the 8.30 meeting of Ward B, Mr. C. had stayed behind and told him that he was worried because Mr. M. had boasted to him that he had taken the £30. This we felt might well be true as it conformed closely to the pattern he had manifested on the occasion of a previous misdemeanour. It was agreed that the psychiatrist should interview Mr. M. immediately before he left hospital.

When seen Mr. M. denied his complicity and was considerably upset at first, but soon reverted to his usual confident and rather cynical self; he departed for his home apparently on good terms with everyone.

In one group the members spontaneously discussed the 9 a.m. meeting, Mr. P. and Mrs. N. both described themselves as 'silent members' and quite frankly admitted that they were afraid of making enemies by verbalizing their thoughts in the 9 a.m. meeting. They then went on to discuss the split in Ward B, but confined themselves to the very narrow topic of the teapot and the anonymous patient who, as leader of the dominant group, shared the tea with half the ward only. This individual (Mr. R.) was named without hesitation in the group and, in the discussion which followed, the group divided itself into his protagonists and his antagonists. No one seemed to consider that the quarrel over the tea might be symptom of a much deeper misunderstanding in the ward.

Another group also chose to lead off by discussing the 9 a.m. meeting. Mr. C., who had originally exposed the split in Ward B and had identified himself with the oppressed ward group, expressed his delight at the immediate effect of the 9 a.m. meeting. Mr. R. (the leader of the dominant group) had sought him out and been very friendly offering him the full facilities of the kitchen, etc. Mr. C. felt that the difficulties in Ward B might well be over, the more so as Mr. M. was leaving that day.

Wednesday 26th March, 8.30 a.m. Meeting

It was decided by the staff that Ward B should again have a meeting in the hope that further information might be forthcoming about the ward tension. Moreover, the patients might discuss certain rumours about a farewell party for Mr. M. in Ward B kitchen on Monday night, the night of the attempted roof burglary by three unidentified men.

During Tuesday the nurses had learnt that Ward B had believed that the nocturnal happenings in their ward were the reason for calling the 8.30 a.m. meeting on Tuesday, and they had been surprised when these happenings were never mentioned. When Ward B assembled they appeared to be in a friendly mood. The psychiatrist asked them why no one had raised the question of the disturbances in the ward during Monday night as they had originally thought that to be the reason for yesterday's ward meeting. Mr. G. said aggressively that if the doctor had asked a question he would have got an answer. The psychiatrist pointed out that the freest possible communication between patients and staff was of great importance if we were to resolve our current Unit problems. At this point the patients began to talk quite freely; some had wakened during the night to see Mr. M. walking through the ward. Then quite spontaneously Mr. T. said that he was one of the culprits and he would give a full statement. He said that along with two other patients he had left the ward after 'lights out' and that they had been on the point of breaking into the canteen when they were observed. The idea was apparently Mr. M.'s who wanted to do something aggressive the night before he was discharged from hospital. Mr. T. felt that they would almost certainly be caught and this somehow made it easier for him to take part, as he wanted to be punished. He then rather reluctantly disclosed the name of Mr. V., the third member of their party. Ward B agreed to continue their discussion at the 9 a.m. meeting and to repeat the story as already known. Mr. T. agreed to this, but wanted to withhold the names of the other two patients. This was, however, rejected by the other patients on the grounds that this was a community, and not a ward problem, and everyone on the Unit had the right to know all the facts.

9 a.m. Meeting

The psychiatrist opened the discussion by explaining why Ward B were being asked to start the discussion for the second successive day instead of having one of the more usual projection techniques such as a sociodrama. He explained that it was now known that Ward B had had a more serious problem yesterday than the tea incident, but had failed to verbalize it. He gave a partial summary of the 8.30 a.m. meeting and a full statement as to why Mr. M. had left hospital on the previous day. Ward B then developed the theme of the ward disturbance on Monday night and Mr. T. repeated his confession; but the other patients demanded more detail and eventually wanted to know the name of the third person involved in the attempted burglary. Mr. V. was present in the audience, but made no move to speak; no one in Ward B seemed inclined to say his name; the doctor broke the awkward pause by saying that it was well known to many people that the third person was Mr. V. and in order to prevent rumour and to lessen the tension he had no hesitation in communicating this knowledge to the rest of the community.

Some patients criticized the staff for not being more strict and allowing patients to slip out of the ward, etc. At this point Mr. F. introduced an apparent irrelevancy by raising his own problem of alcoholism. He compared this 'minor' crime with the 'major' crime of attempted theft by Mr. T. He stressed the fact that his drunkenness in the Unit was a symptom of his illness which resulted from unhappiness and suggested that the staff should be more liberal in their attitude towards his behaviour than they had been. The psychiatrist suggested that this was a separate topic and might be discussed further at another meeting. But Mr. F. was not to be placated and announced his intention to discharge himself before he was asked to leave. The group adopted a supportive attitude and urged him to stay.

The discussion then reverted to the attempted burglary and Mr. T. came in for a considerable amount of criticism. However, other patients tried to find motives to explain the misdemeanour. The psychiatrist pointed out that as three different people were involved they might well have three quite different motives. As an illustration he described the type of person who would participàte in such an escapade in the hope of being caught and punished. The group seemed to accept this possibility of complex individual motivations in such a situation. The psychiatrist then continued to elaborate on the current situation and how the community's problem had been considerably eased by the morning's events. It was now a matter for each patient concerned to be treated in whatever way his own doctor thought best. The meeting had lasted eighty minutes and had been held in an atmosphere highly charged with emotion throughout; nevertheless towards the end there seemed to be a feeling of uniformity and goodwill.

9.45 a.m. Meeting

The staff felt that there had been an enormous relief of tension during the 9 a.m. meeting, and that it had been wise to prolong the meeting so that the problem could be adequately worked through. The discharge of Mr. M. on the day previous to the confession of Mr. T. had removed much of the fear and uncertainty which had blocked communication and had undermined the patients' confidence in the staff. It was felt that although the patients had to some extent come to accept that theft and other antisocial behaviour were symptoms of an illness, they nevertheless needed to feel that the staff were strong enough to protect them if need be. It had needed the demonstration of this protection by discharging Mr. M. to allow the patient population to play a more active community role. It was felt that Mr. M. had been largely responsible for the participation of the other two culprits and as the latter were psychiatrically very ill their antisocial conduct should be considered as part of their illnesses and dealt with accordingly. It was still not quite certain who had stolen the £30, but there was every reason to suspect Mr. M.

In one therapeutic group the members felt that the 9 a.m. meeting was the most interesting one that they had ever attended. Four patients, all women, went further and said that it had given them an insight into the organization and principles of the Unit which they had lacked previously. They identified themselves closely with the staff attitude towards social problems, punishment and informing. The fact that no one was punished had surprised and impressed them, despite repeated staff assurances in the past that no punishment was contemplated. However, two male patients seemed to have learnt nothing. They were apparently quite unaware of the social growth which had occurred in certain sections of the Unit community and they still clung on to their 'schoolboyish' attitude towards informing in the case of antisocial behaviour.

Another group also talked spontaneously about the 9 a.m. meeting. Five members expressed ideas which showed a close identification with the staff attitude towards social problems, communication and punishment, but two patients said that they had been in the Unit too short a time (two and nine days respectively) to fully understand what was going on. Another patient, while agreeing that there had been a tremendous change in community attitudes in recent weeks, felt that the factors contributing to this change might prove to be much more complex than the immediate discussion indicated.

The above account has been given in some detail in order to illustrate the planning and form of our community meetings. The staff attempts to achieve general agreement in relation to current social problems, and their attitude is made known to the patient population through the social therapy techniques. The patients are afforded numerous opportunities for the expression or acting out of emotional difficulties in a group setting. According to circumstance, these are handled spontaneously or follow a predetermined pattern. We attempt to plan the social structure of the Unit in such a way that free communication is obtained and maintained between all members of the community.

During the ten days covered by this report the social problems of theft, discipline and informing were all dealt with in the way described. Certain changes towards these problems seemed to occur in at least some members of the community. The staff also was involved in this process of change, and it is felt that as the more permanent members of the population, they now act as carriers of this cultural change. Clearly there are many factors involved other than those described. One extraneous factor which almost certainly contributed to the change of social climate was the discharge of Mr. M. The removal of this frightening influence appears to have made it possible for silent members to speak in group and community meetings, and also reassured the patient population that although the staff aim was essentially therapeutic, they could also play a protective role when needed.

In conclusion, full details of the original theft of £30 were provided by Mr. V. who confessed his own part in this and confirmed our suspicions regarding Mr. M. He admitted to a long history of delinquency which he had never been able to discuss before. He felt that our insistence on stealing being a symptom had given him a different attitude to himself and his behaviour, and made confession possible. He said that he had often wanted to confess both to his family and to others, but he had been unable to do so. He would have confessed earlier, but felt some loyalty to Mr. M., and could not do so until he had gone. It is of interest that one week after Mr. V.'s confession, he told his doctor that he had expected to be discharged, in spite of our repeated assurances to the contrary. He now felt sufficiently secure to discuss his current problems with his father in a way which he had never been able to do previously.

The Unit culture is a constantly changing one. It is realized that the attitudes adopted towards theft and informing as described in this addendum, are controversial and only further experience can confirm or disprove their value.

INDEX

185

Printed and bound by CPI Group (UK) Ltd, Croydon, CR0 4YY

01/11/2024

01782629-0003